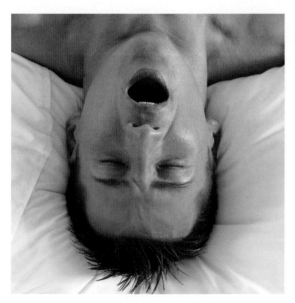

DRIVE HIM WILD
100 sex tips for women

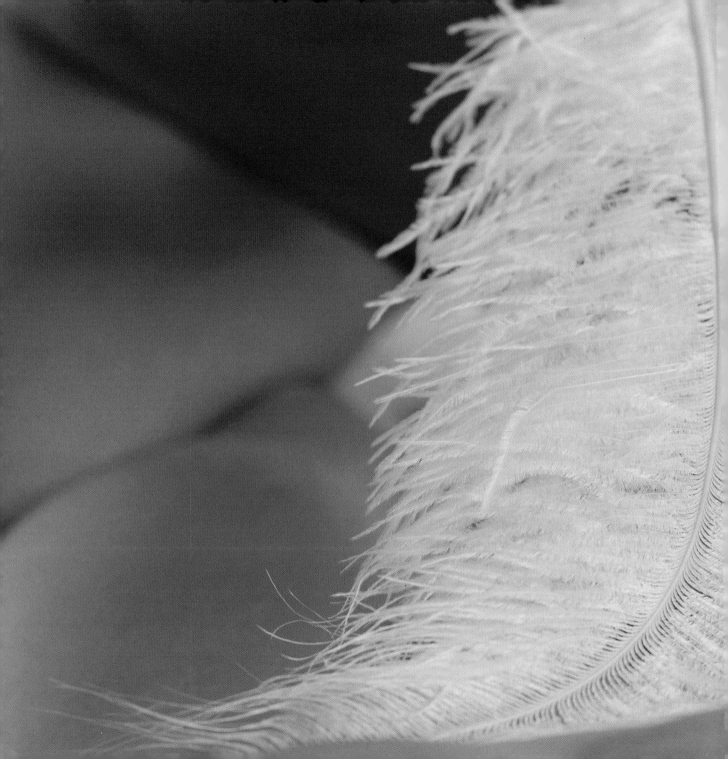

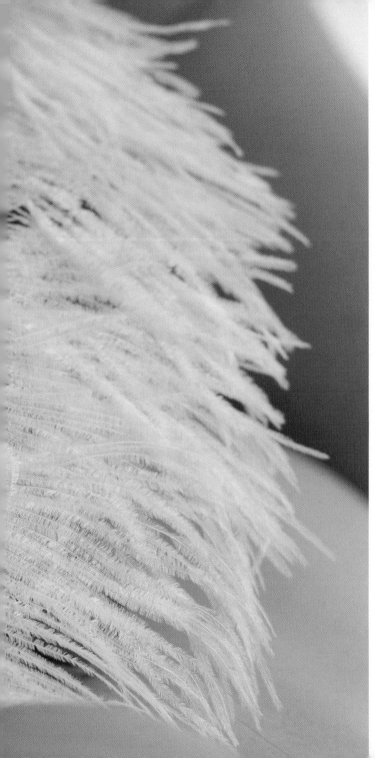

DRIVE HIM WILD
100 sex tips for women

Katy Bevan

Photography by John Freeman

LORENZ BOOKS

This edition is published by Lorenz Books,
an imprint of Anness Publishing Ltd, Blaby Road, Wigston,
Leicestershire LE18 4SE; info@anness.com

www.lorenzbooks.com; www.annesspublishing.com

If you like the images in this book and would like to investigate
using them for publishing, promotions or advertising, please visit
our website www.practicalpictures.com for more information.

Publisher – Joanna Lorenz
Project Editor – Katy Bevan
Copy Editor – Alison Bolus
Designer – PB Wagon for RB-M Studio
Photography – John Freeman assisted by Alex Dow
Hair and Make-up – Bettina Graham
Production Controller – Steve Lang

© Anness Publishing Ltd 2013

A CIP catalogue record for this book is available from
the British Library.

PUBLISHER'S NOTE
Although the advice and information in this book are believed to be
accurate and true at the time of going to press, neither the authors
nor the publisher can accept any legal responsibility or liability for
any errors or omissions that may have been made nor for any
inaccuracies nor for any loss, harm or injury that comes about from
following instructions or advice in this book.

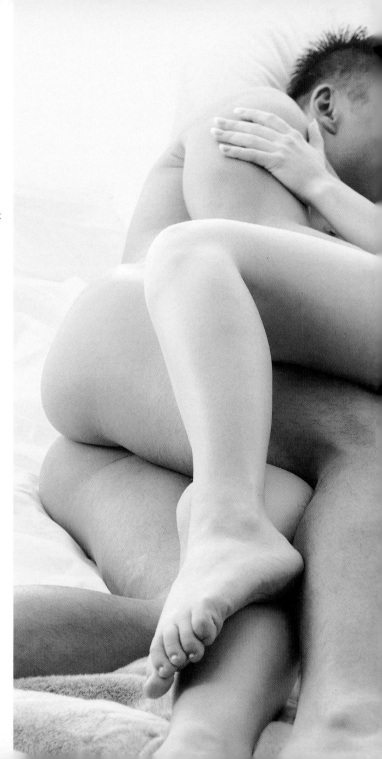

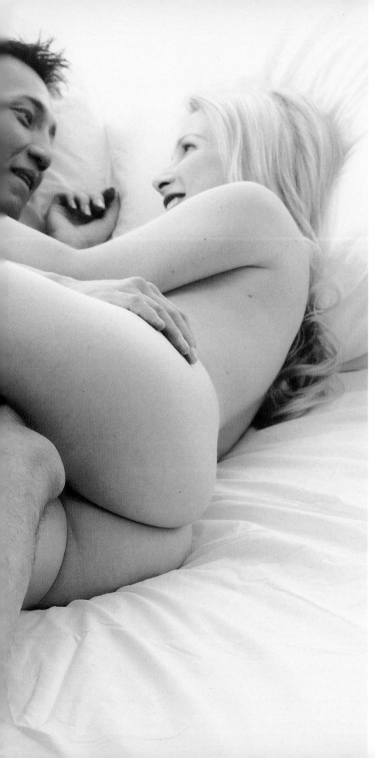

Contents

Introduction 7

1 Anticipation
Techniques for seduction 10
10 ways to kiss him..12
10 places to touch him 14
Foreplay to please him 17
10 tips for fabulous foreplay..18

2 Every which way
Positions for sex 22
10 positions to amaze him 24
10 top places for great sex 28

3 The big O
Orgasm..32
10 tips for the ultimate orgasm 34
10 hot toys and how to use them… 36

4 Going down
What every woman should know about oral sex 40
10 hot tips for fantastic fellatio..42

5 Divine inspiration
Ancient erotica 48
Tips from the Ananga Ranga 50
10 tips for exotic sex..52

6 Making it even better
Pushing the boundaries..56
10 ways to spice it up..58
What every woman should know about contraception 62

Index 64

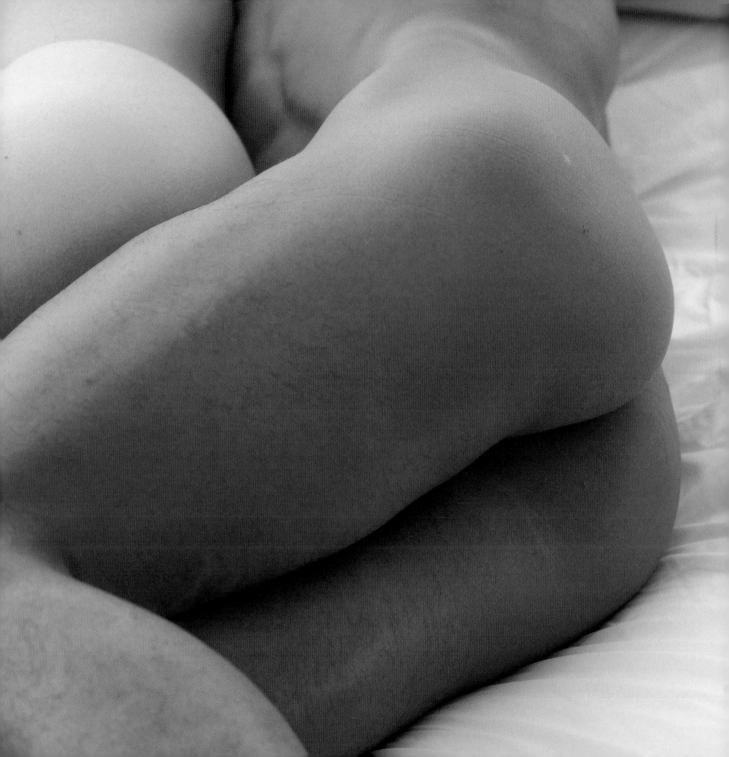

...The art of making love is to give, give, give, while being very sure that you are going to get what you need in return...

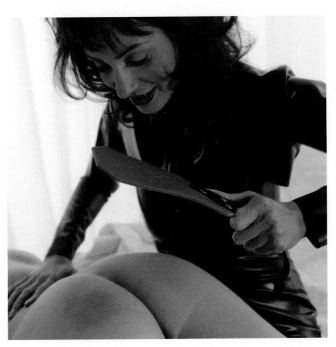

Introduction

You have made your catch – the niceties are over, so what do you do now? This little book will give you enough tips to continue with panache to the finishing line, rather than being left standing, clueless, at the starting post. It's not just the first-timers that need encouragement – couples who have been together for years can get stuck in a boring-sex routine that it is hard to break. This book will give you the inspiration and confidence to try things you have never attempted before, and amaze your man.

So now you have him in the sack, what do you do with him? Why isn't he doing all the gorgeous things to you that you have imagined? Rather than making your demands with a blackboard and a piece of chalk, one approach is to give him what he wants, in the manner you would like it returned to you. Get the picture? All that selfless massaging in the wee small hours might pay back huge dividends in the long run. And, let's face it, if it doesn't, he'll be out on his ear anyway.

You shouldn't feel that you have to do anything that you don't want to do. But, on the other hand, if you are expecting him to go down on you, for instance, and all the luxury that entails for you, you might feel it is only fair to reciprocate. Still, as they say, "all's fair in love", which means, of course, that it is no such thing. What you give will definitely not be what you get in this game, so forget that from the start. Somewhere along the line a balance needs to be achieved that is satisfactory to all concerned. The art of making love is to give, give, give, while being very sure that you are going to get what you need in return. For men, this is usually quite straightforward, as they think they know exactly what they want, or need. For women, it is a little more complicated. Generally speaking, you know what you are going to get, but the trick is to make sure that it happens in the way you want.

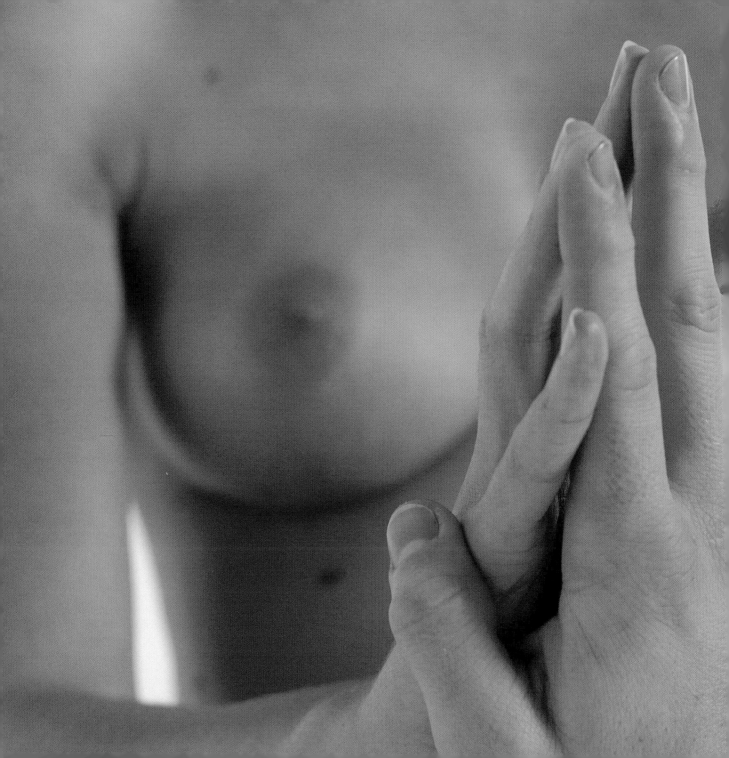

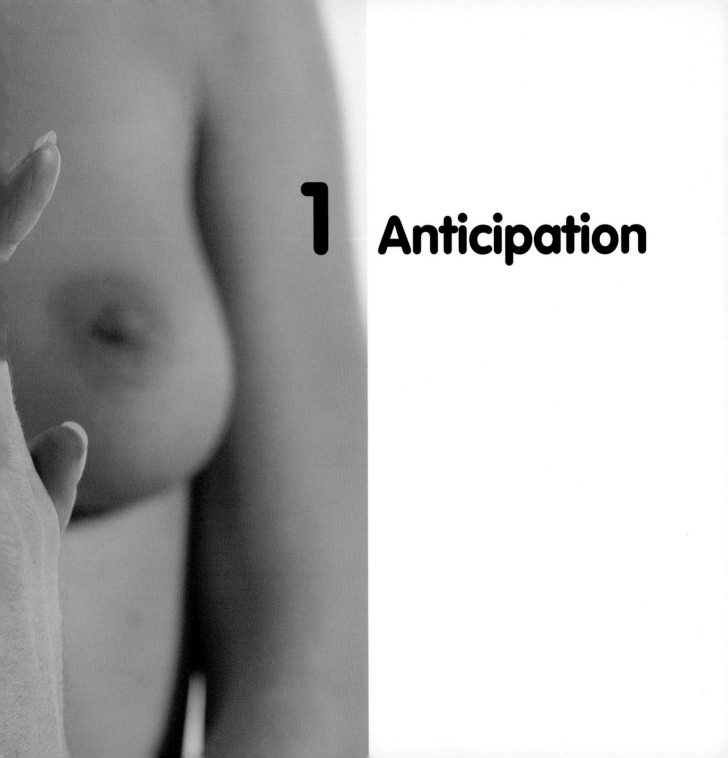

1 Anticipation

...You may not have really touched him before, so this is where to make your mark as Ms Irresistible...

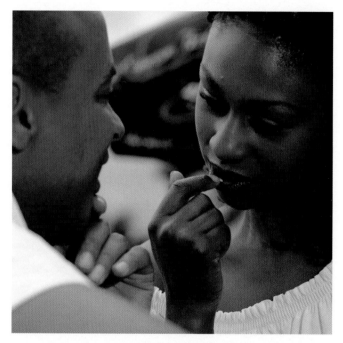

Techniques for seduction

It is all in the anticipation – the longer the build-up to sex, the better the crescendo when you finally arrive. This is about seduction in the broadest sense. We are assuming that you have already made your conquest. You have enjoyed those lingering looks over the coffee machine, and those tantalizing brushes of the arm. Now we get down to the serious bit in private.

You may not have really touched him before, so this is where to make your mark as Ms Irresistible. Radiating confidence is the best way to ensure that you are attractive to him. Think sexy, potent goddess, and that is what you will project. The mind is a powerful organ and will help you to overcome any hang-ups you may have about your ability or your body. Forget trying to imitate anyone else – the strength you have is your uniqueness. No one will touch him in the same way that you do, and no one else will respond to his touch in the same way that you do. Concentration is the key if you are nervous, or even bored by the whole idea – focus completely on him, and you will become his personal sex goddess.

Oral caressing

Kissing can set the pace for the type of lovemaking you want to indulge in. Try a slow, loving kiss, caressing his mouth with your tongue, or a more passionate, frenzied kiss, where you are slightly rougher and more urgent with each other. Small kisses all over your lover's body will make him go wild with desire.

Most people like the idea of kissing someone with smooth and shapely lips, a generous smile and good teeth. Bad teeth are one of the ultimate turn-offs. Lip size doesn't indicate whether someone is a good kisser or not, but some mouths are just so kissable. It could be the shape, the smile or the fullness of the lips, or even the way the person wets their lips with their tongue.

A survey carried out on kissing showed that women like kissing better than men and enjoy the whole long, lingering embrace without it necessarily leading to anything else. In fact, some women have said that they find kissing the most erotic part of sex, and have often had an orgasm just from a passionate session of kissing. Most men will be able to take it or leave it, so it is your job to show him how fantastic an oral caress can be.

Apart from the mouth and cheeks, there are loads of other places on his body that are just begging to be kissed – eyelids, nose, ears, neck (delicious), armpits (yes, really), insides of wrists, fingertips, backs of knees, ankles, soles and toes, and lots more places in between. The best way to find out his favourite places is to go on a kissing tour of your lover, working your way around his whole body.

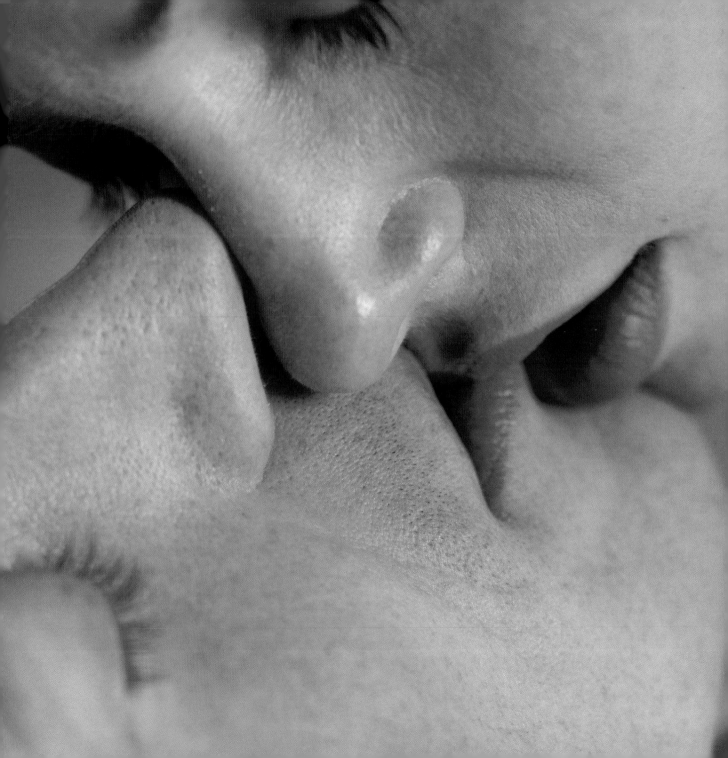

10 ways to kiss him

The truth is that men aren't into kissing half as much as women are. That said, they will enjoy it more if you take the lead. Why not show him the way that you would like to be kissed by doing it to him first? He may pick up some hints. The ideas given here are just for starters. Once you get into your stride, you can invent any kind of oral caress that seems to work for him.

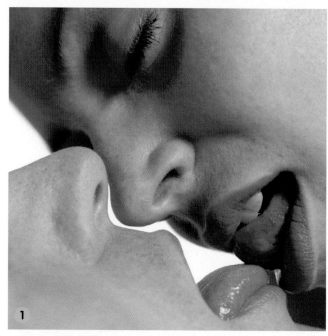

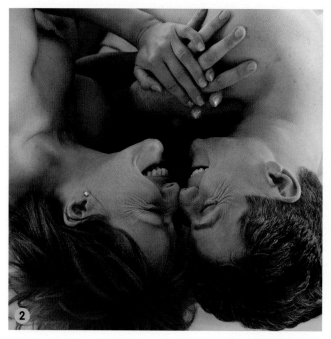

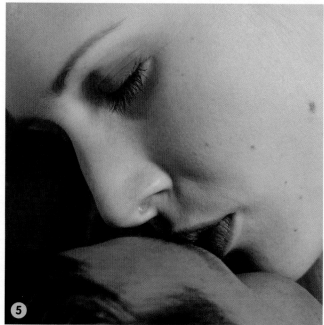

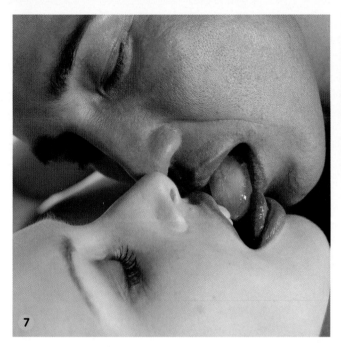

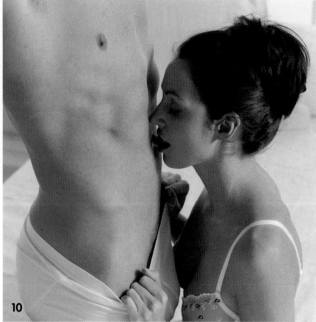

1 French kissing
You really should have mastered the basic snog by this stage of the game. First of all you need to relax, tip your head to one side to avoid nose collisions, and let your lips touch his. Once you have established contact, you can initiate some further action, such as touching tongues. Then gently caress the inside of your partner's mouth with your tongue. As he responds, you can quicken the pace and intensity, going for a fuller thrust.

2 Rubbing noses
This type of greeting, often called 'Eskimo' kissing, is associated with the Inuit and with Pacific islanders. Each person literally inhales the odour of the other person. Animals do it all the time.

3 Silent but deadly
Some of the sexiest kisses are the silent ones, lips and eyes closed, while caressing his hair, face and neck with your hands.

4 Stereophonic kiss
Moan or slurp while you're kissing. Some people adore the sound and sensation of the inside of their ears being kissed – the sloshing sound really turns them on.

5 Wandering kiss
Hold your partner's face between your hands and kiss different parts of his face, first each eyebrow, then eyelids, nose and so on, and between each kiss say something erotic. Describe what you are going to do to him, how you want him to kiss or lick you, where, and what position you want to try. What you say depends on how dirty you want to be.

6 Nibbling
Don't bite: it hurts. Love bites are not clever. Nuzzling, on the other hand, is delightful. Take his bottom lip gently between your teeth and tug on it, being careful not to take part of him with you. Nibbling is also good for any part of his body that stays still long enough.

7 Ice games
If he is playing hard-to-get, ask him to retrieve an ice-cube from your lips. The challenge is to keep it moving between you without using your hands. Of course, the ice will eventually melt away, and that is when the game really begins.

8 Butterfly kiss
Tried and tested. Use your eyelashes to brush against his face or body.

9 Finger kissing
Get your digits in on the action and into his mouth. The different texture and pace will definitely spice things up.

10 Detour
This could be for anything up to 2 minutes, but don't leave it too long, or you will both have forgotten what you were doing. The ears, the navel and the top of his spine are all places worth the journey.

10 places to touch him

Don't feel that you always have to be soft and gentle. Men sometimes like a bit of rough and tumble, though don't forget that your aim is to relax and arouse, not to hurt or irritate. Some men are not very tactile creatures, and may need to be encouraged, and some men think that any touching will lead straight to intercourse. This is where you need to step in and take control, to show him how affectionate caresses can be a pleasure in their own right, not just a means to an end.

Try not to go straight for his genitals, but explore other parts of his body – fingers, toes, armpits and navel – first. Really tantalize each other with massaging hand strokes followed by tender licks and kisses, and then one thing can lead to another, if you are ready.

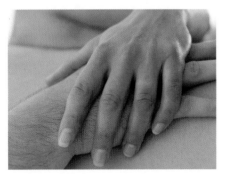

1 Navel

The skin around the navel is much thinner than elsewhere, making it an extremely sensitive area. Navels have taken on a new lease of life since they have begun to be decorated with tattoos and navel rings or studs, and displayed above low-slung jeans. Some people are a bit squeamish about their navels, but others enjoy having them caressed by a soft tongue. It may make them giggle a bit, but, after all, this is meant to be fun.

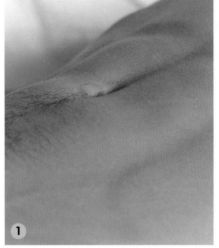

2 Toe job

This is one of those things men either love or hate. Some people find the idea of placing a set of toes anywhere near their lips revolting, whereas others find it a real turn-on. If cleanliness is an issue for you, then why not treat your partner to a pre-toe job pedicure? Providing he is not too ticklish, the pedicure process can be very relaxing. Alternatively, encourage him to have a bath and a good scrub beforehand, and then moisturize his feet. You'll find feet can be a seriously sexy zone once you start to take care of them. It will start to look as if all those foot fetishists can't be wrong.

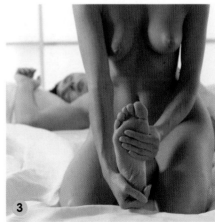

3 Insteps

For those who can manage to have their feet touched without collapsing in hysterics, the instep of the foot is a sensitive, nerve-rich area that can be licked and stroked. Many people love to have their feet massaged and pampered, and the feet can also be used as an interesting and different way to stimulate other areas of the body – but make sure they're warmed up first.

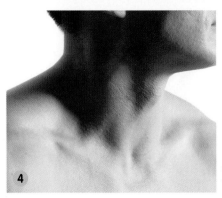

4 Nape of the neck

There is something strangely comforting and at the same time sensually delightful about having the back of your neck stroked. It sends a mixture of warmth and thrilling shock waves along the entire length of your spine, leaving you feeling energized and loved. This is a very relaxing and loving place to caress your partner, as it has a mysterious link to his sensual centre.

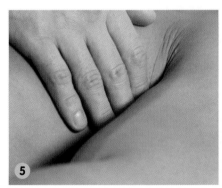

5 Armpits

No one is suggesting that you bury your face in your partner's armpits just as he leaves the gym, but think just how sensitive your armpits are. They are a veritable minefield of nerve endings, and after a bath or shower they respond well to some gentle caressing and tingling licks.

6 Fingers

The fingers are an understandably popular focus of attention, not least because the tips are so sensitive. During a romantic meal, you may feed each other, licking and sucking the juices from fingers and wrists. The act of sucking fingers is very erotic because it is loaded with innuendo.

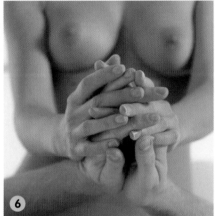

7 Bottom

This area is so gorgeously irresistible that it will be hard to stop yourself taking a bite. He will love it, too, if you make a fuss of his pert derrière (if he has one, that is).

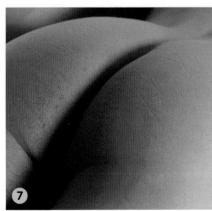

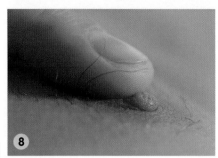

8 Nipples

Men love to have their nipples tantalizingly tickled. They, too, have hundreds of nerve endings here, and the nipples get erect and stiff, much like your own. Try a gentle rotating touch, running circles around the nipple area, and tousling any hairs en route.

9 Ears

Well, you could be whispering sweet nothings, but you might have more effect if you gently nibble his ear lobes. Some men adore the swishing sounds of a full-on tongue-quest for the full aural experience.

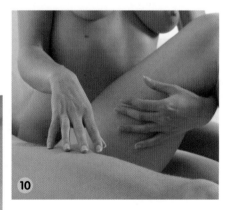

10 Thighs

This will drive him wild. You have been on a tour around his body, steadfastly ignoring his genitals, and now you are inching closer. Once you have been here, it would be cruel not to continue any farther.

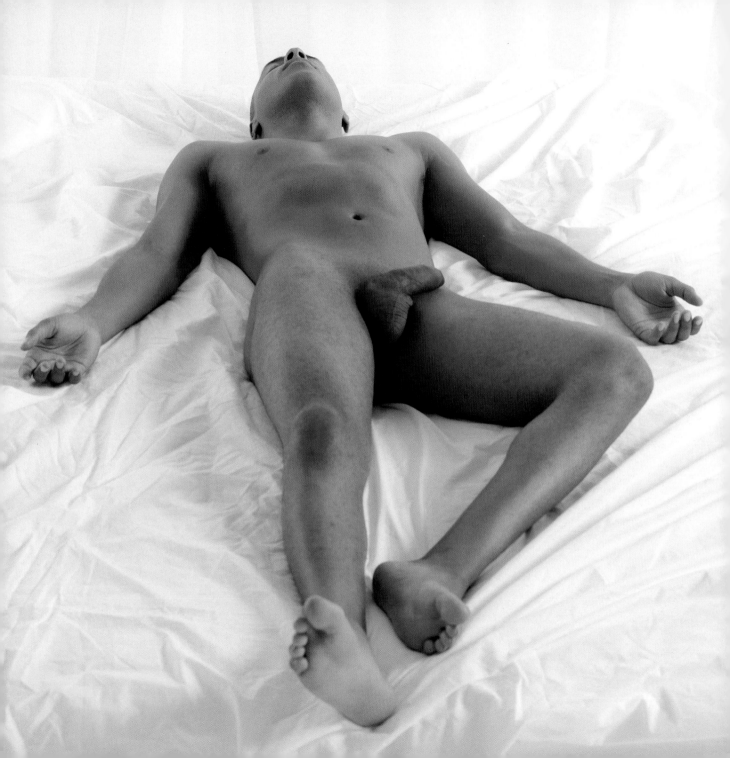

...most men claim to be bored silly by the whole idea – but foreplay is for men too...

Foreplay to please him

Okay, so we all know that women favour a long and drawn-out session of foreplay, and that most men claim to be bored silly by the whole idea – but foreplay is for men too.

Since 95 per cent of men masturbate, they will know what to expect. But being touched by someone else can be completely different. Have you ever tried to tickle yourself? Then you'll know what I mean. It is important that men get up to sexual speed, as this will result in a more intense orgasm.

So where do you begin? Instead of concentrating solely on the penis, try to explore other areas, such as his nipples, chest, thighs, perineum and buttocks. Gradually get closer to your goal, and he will be going wild with anticipation.

There is no right or wrong way to stimulate a man's penis. Some men prefer a strong, gripping movement, others enjoy a lighter touch. Many men prefer to confine stimulation to the head or glans alone. This may involve a pulling action, which stimulates just the head and frenulum area. Other men incorporate the shaft into their technique.

Finally, if you have never tried stimulating his anus, give it a go. Whatever works, wins.

Biology lesson

Understanding more about the structure of the important parts of the male body is a great start to improving your lovemaking skills. In spite of the apparent complexity and perplexity of its character, the penis is a remarkably simple organ in both structure and function.

The head, or glans, is the mushroom-shaped part at the end of the shaft, and this is the end point for a lot of nerves, making it one of the most sensitive areas. In the uncircumcised man, the flaccid penis is covered with a thin membranous layer of skin called the prepuce, or foreskin. When an uncircumcised man gets hard, this

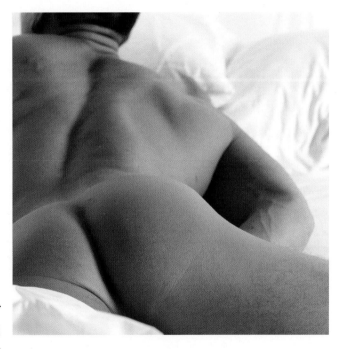

layer of skin slips back to display the glans, and during sex it retracts further, so that the glans is fully exposed.

The frenulum is located on the underside of the penis, where the head meets the shaft in a puckering and folding of skin that tethers the foreskin to the head. It is an area of particular sensitivity, so it should never be ignored during lovemaking.

The corona is the ridge around the base of the glans where it meets the shaft. It is so sensitive that some say that light pressure around it can suppress orgasm and lengthen lovemaking.

The perineum is the area of sensitive skin that covers the stretch between the anus and the testicles. This is a miniature playground of pleasure, complete with its own delicious mixture of nerve endings and hot spots offering endless possibilities.

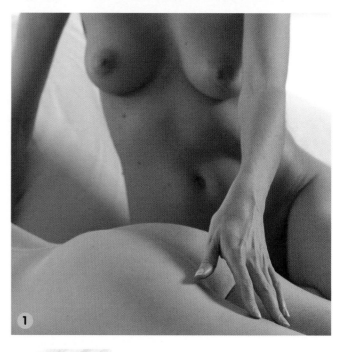

10 tips for fabulous foreplay

The techniques described here have been tried and tested. They are merely a guide, however, as you will soon find what pleases your man, and then you can elaborate on that. Use a firm touch – his penis is quite different from any part of your body. Once he has discovered the heights of passion he can reach with foreplay, he'll be converted for life.

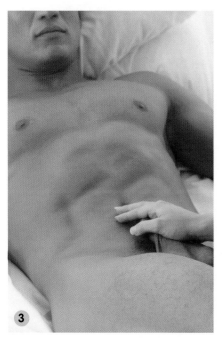

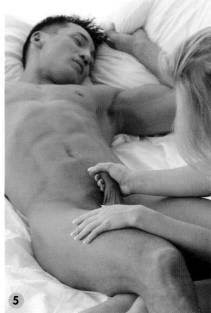

1 Explore

First of all, explore his body and familiarize yourself with it. Have a little self-guided tour, so that you have a mental body map before you begin in earnest. He is sure not to object.

2 Lubrication

For some men, lubrication won't be a necessary part of foreplay, but since it changes the sensations you create, why not give it a go? Water-based lubricants are best, and there are several on the market, but don't choose one with a spermicide, as it will taste revolting if some gets near your mouth.

3 Rising dough

If he is lying on his back and not showing any signs of arousal, press his penis against his stomach with the palm of your hand and knead it as if it were dough – he'll be rising in no time. Form two rings around the penis with the thumb and forefinger of each hand, and try pulling them in opposite directions.

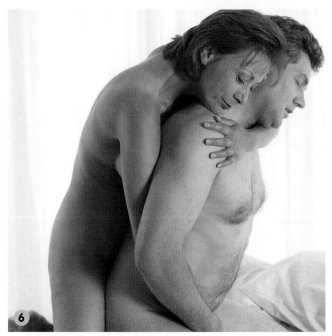
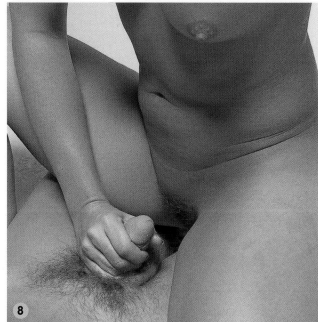

4 Testicle tantalizer
Hold his testicles in your hand and squeeze gently, without making any strong or jerky movements. With the tips of your fingers or with your other hand, you can stroke his perineum, the sensitive area between the testes and his anus. This will send waves of pleasure through his body.

5 Calligraphy grip
Hold his penis in the way that you would a pen. Stroke his penis up and down in this way, stimulating the frenulum and glans. If he needs more contact, simply wrap the rest of your fingers around to form a fist, and use your thumb at the top to stimulate the head.

6 Turn and twist
Sitting behind him, grip the top of the head like a water tap and twist as you would if turning a tap on or off. This may be better with some lubrication and stimulation of the shaft with your other hand.

7 Prayer pumper
Put your hands tightly together as if in prayer. Add some lubrication, and then ask him to insert his penis into the groove formed at the joining of your wrists. Once he gets the idea, he can thrust into your hands, adjusting the depth of penetration.

8 San Francisco shuffle
Hold his penis in a similar way to the calligraphy grip, using either a fist or your thumb and forefinger. Stroke up and then, instead of going straight back down, go over the top of the head, maintaining contact, then twist your hand, and come down again with the top of your hand closest to his stomach and your thumb pointing away from the body. Then reverse the direction.

9 Dressing up
For this one, all you need to do is experiment with different fabrics and textures, by placing socks, gloves and other garments over his penis. Different fabrics will provide a variety of sensations. The cool chill of silk, for example, will induce a sensation similar to water, whereas the harder, rougher and warmer feel of leather, combined with its distinctive smell, is a completely different sensory experience. Experimentation is the key here, and soon you will become more aware of which textures turn him on.

10 Anal probe
He might not be sure about this one at first, but is sure to become a convert. While you are stroking his perineum, try to gently caress his anus. The area around the anus is one of the most sensitive parts of his body, and so a potential source of sensory possibilities. This is the gateway to his prostate gland, or G-spot – the playground for many a happy hour of exploration. Try licking your smallest finger and seeing if you can insert it there. If he flinches, don't be offended, perhaps just try again later.

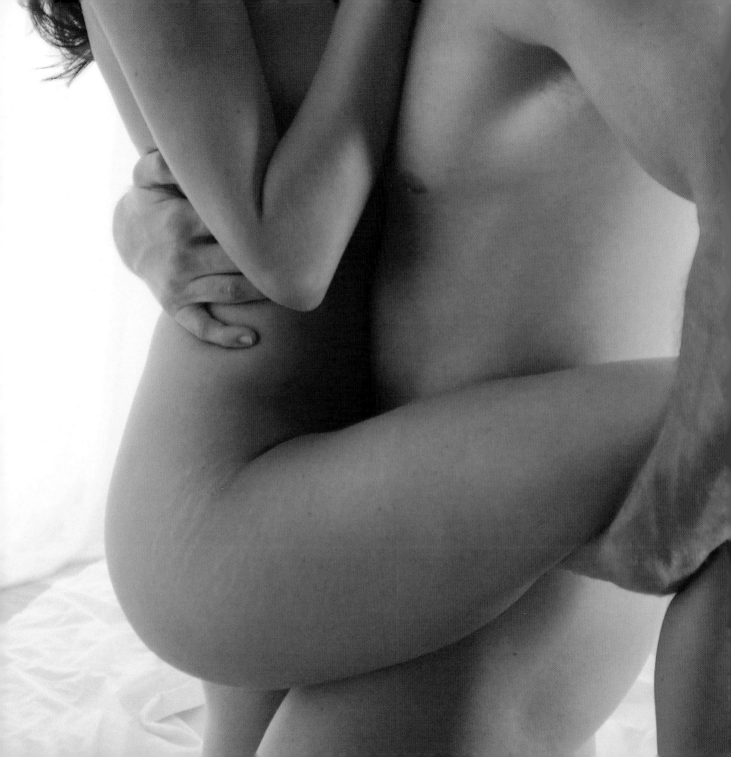

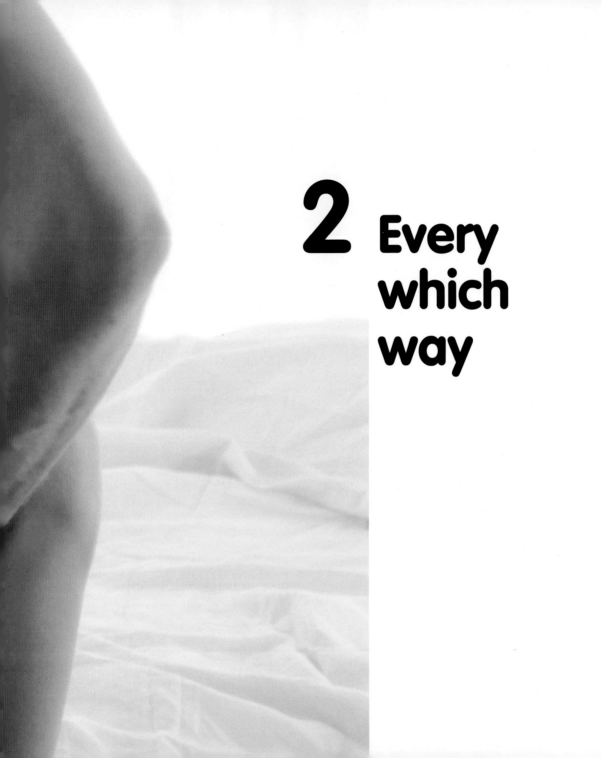

2 Every which way

…what men really like is the visual feast – an eyeful of what they fancy really does turn them on…

Positions for sex

Sex is a two-person game (on most weekdays, anyway), and the trick here is to make sure you both get what you want. The majority of women don't orgasm through penetration alone, so it is in your interest to choose positions that not only please your partner but also maximize clitoral contact. The position of the clitoris varies between women, and those who have theirs nearer the vagina will be more easily stimulated. For the rest of us, there are ways of ensuring that at least part of him is in contact with the clitoris or the other sensitive tissue around the labia.

Everyone has an opinion and preference on sexual positions, and although it is unwise to generalize, there are some that men like more than others. Some are spoons subscribers, while others are doggy devotees, but what men really like is the visual feast – an eyeful of what they fancy really does turn them on.

Men will love to have you climb on top and take the reins. It is often the shy, quiet women who turn out to be trumps at this game, and the domineering men who are itching to be told what to do. Take charge of the situation and get on top – he'll go wild for the full-frontal view. He even gets to watch his penis go in and out.

It is also true that men love to go doggy-style. This isn't every girl's favourite position, as there is a dearth of eye contact, and kissing is tricky. Try not to get a crick in the neck, just give in to it. He will love the extra-deep penetration and the posterior vantage point, and, if you have your hands free, you can stimulate his testicles and stroke his perineum, making this position an absolute winner for him.

Ringing the changes
It certainly makes for a more interesting sex life if you vary your positions, and, although this doesn't need to be done with military precision, it can be great fun experimenting with something new.

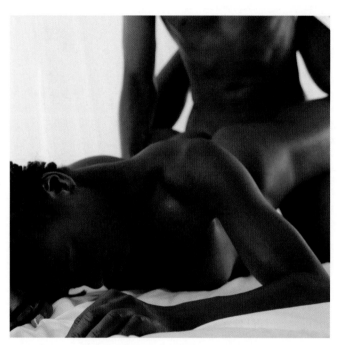

All it takes is a little imagination, practice and enthusiasm (and, at times, the magic ingredient – humour).

Physical and verbal communication with your partner are both paramount. As you learn his likes and dislikes, you'll be able to anticipate when to change positions or when to lead. He'll find it a great turn-on if you suggest a new position, saying, "I've read about this one. Shall we give it a go?"

Most of us are creatures of habit and usually opt for only two or three sexual positions because they are tried-and-tested favourites. But familiarity leads to bedroom boredom, and this is to be avoided. Trying new positions may seem strange at first, but it really does add spice to your sex life, and, once you have opened the door on some experimentation, he may surprise you with some tricks of his own.

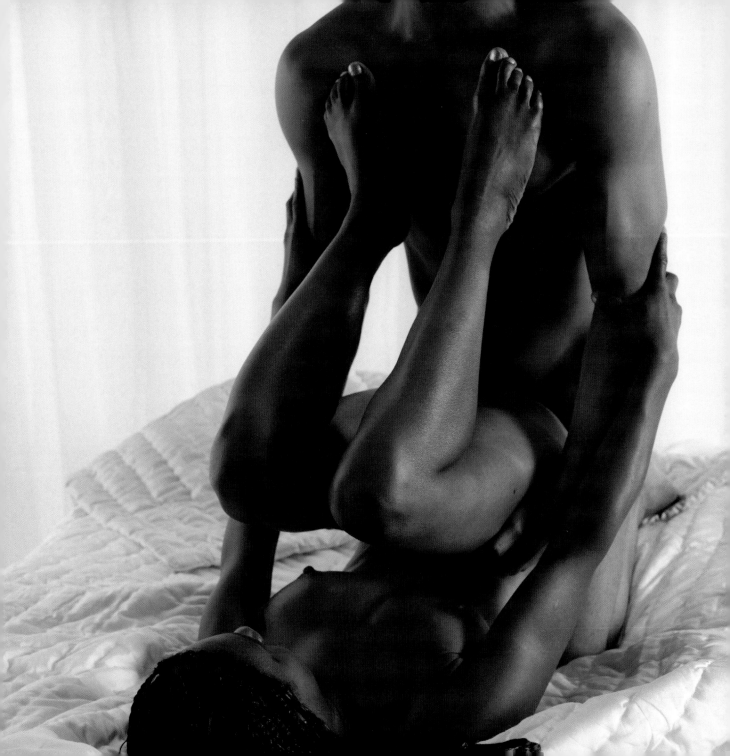

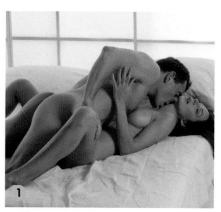

1

10 positions to amaze him

For really good sex you need to have a repertoire of different positions to keep your lovemaking interesting, stimulating and truly satisfying. Although more than 600 sexual postures have been recorded – some very weird and wonderful – most of them in fact stem from six basic positions. You may think that you have tried them all before, but here are some extra tips to help you drive him into a frenzy. He won't want to have sex in the same position every time, any more than you do, but may be scared to try something new. This is where you can be assertive and show him a thing or two. He will definitely thank you for the trouble.

There is no denying that some positions work very well, which is why we are tempted to come back to them again and again. However, even the most exciting positions can suffer from repetition, and it is always a good idea to have something else you can produce spontaneously, to enliven a dull evening at the drop of a hat.

Men and women both want the same thing – he wants increased sensation, and so do you. However, you both need stimulation in different areas, so that's the balancing trick to learn. Once you do, it will keep you both smiling.

1 Him on top

You have tried to interest him in some new positions, but inevitably you end up with that old faithful – the missionary (that's the one where you get squashed underneath him). But there are some things you can do to improve the situation.

To make it more interesting for him, caress his testicles and the shaft of his penis before he enters you. Once he's inside, stroke his chest, then work your way down his back with your hands to play with his anus.

On a selfish front, this position is not so good for clitoral stimulation, because the penis is often not at the best angle. But if you arch your back, he can penetrate even deeper. Try placing a pillow under your bottom and bending your legs – you may have to try different angles to get this perfect, but you should find that you can get some friction on your G spot.

2 Him on top with bells on

Okay, so he's still on top. Now wrap your legs around his waist, and pull him inside you. Because of the angle of penetration, even a man who believes his penis is small will feel like a stud. If you are not getting enough stimulation, try doing it for yourself: he'll love watching and may even join in. From here you can pull your knees up to your chest, with one or both feet resting on

his shoulders. If you press your hand on your stomach, you may be able to feel his penis as it moves in and out.

To increase the friction for him, grip your legs together to make the vagina feel tighter. This is where all those pelvic floor muscles come in. Rhythmic squeezing of the vaginal walls will make him wild with passion. If you are really fed up with being squashed underneath, then you may be able to rock him over on to his back, and take charge.

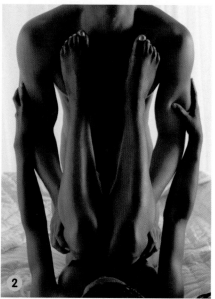

2

3 Climb on board

One of the most common male fantasies is of being dominated by a woman, so why not indulge him and get on top? Some of the most erotic positions are played out here. You are in charge now, and he can only watch you perform. The visual stimulation is great for him, so for men who tend to come too quickly, you may have to slow the pace accordingly.

Climb on top, facing him, with your legs pulled up slightly, so you have freedom of movement. Once he is aroused – and he

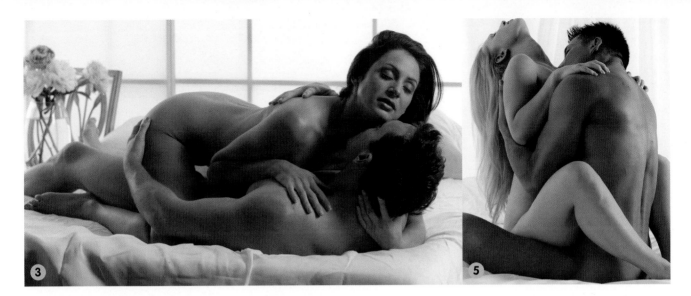

probably will be already – guide his penis inside you before lying down on his chest. Contract your vaginal muscles around his penis, and he will be in heaven. Try pausing at the top of the penis as he comes out, and touch the end of his member at the entrance to the vagina to give him a tantalizing sense of anticipation.

There is no pressure for the man to "perform", and he can enjoy feeling especially loved, while you have control of your own arousal, as well as his. Some men dislike not being in control, but they can usually be persuaded once they have given it a go.

4 Rodeo ride
When you are straddling your man, facing him, you can massage his chest, bend over to lick his nipples and upper body, rock back and forth, and go around and around with your hips. Touch your clitoris at the same time, if you can balance and your legs are strong enough. You can also lean back and grab his ankles for stability. If you get tired, ask him to bend his knees so that you can lean back and take a break. Now comes the *pièce de résistance*.

Slowly turn around, while he is still inside you, keeping your thighs together as much as possible, and you'll be sitting half way around. Then take it all the way and turn so that you are facing the other way. He will love the view from here, though you just get to see his feet. He will be able to gyrate his hips now, which is just as well since you will be exhausted. Lean forwards and try to stay on the bucking bronco you have aroused.

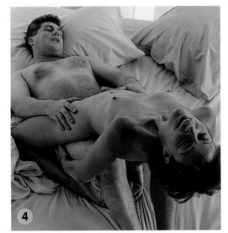

This position is both highly tactile and visually stimulating. It's a fabulous way to indulge all your basic instincts and to demonstrate your feelings for your lover. Penetration is very deep, so it is great for most men and for those women who particularly like that.

5 Full frontal hugging
This is a really intimate position, a little like giving each other an extra-special hug. Sit on his lap, facing him – your legs wrapped around his back. Initially, if you sit slightly away from your partner, you can stroke his penis. When you are both ready, guide him inside, then rock your way to an orgasm.

If you can bear to stop hugging each other, try leaning back and holding each other's hands or arms to help keep you in time. You will be able to tease each other by looking, as you can't touch. Visual stimulation scores highly for both partners when you lean back, and the hands-off effect is really tantalizing. You will also have the added thrill of seeing his penis thrusting in and out. It can take practice to work out the rhythm – but this shouldn't prove too much of a hardship.

6 The hip rotator

You will be more in control with this one. Sit on his lap again, on the floor or a chair. If you place your feet flat, you can easily push yourself up and down. Rotating your hips and making circular motions should drive him wild, as well as being excellent for clitoral stimulation. If you are on the floor, raise yourself up with your legs and pause momentarily, then go down on to his tip and come up again before he has entered you.

You can let him thrust upwards at the same time, but it may take a while to get the timing right together. Since penetration will be quite shallow, experiment with the angles. You can also explore his upper body with your tongue, and, if you are lucky, you might get some reciprocal action. This is a lovely position for hugging, kissing and full body contact.

This is great position in any situation for you and for him – from the garden to the office, on a chair or on the floor. If your legs are short, then that's what the rungs of the chair were made for. Why not try placing the chair in front of a mirror, so that you can watch yourselves? Some people find this very erotic.

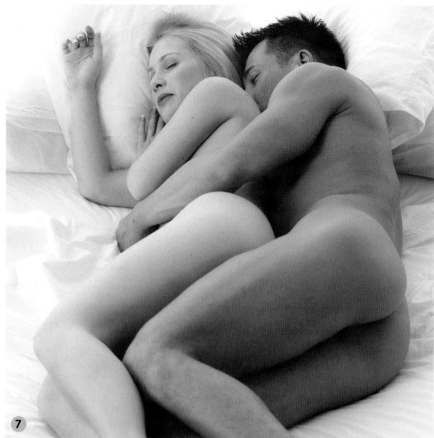

7

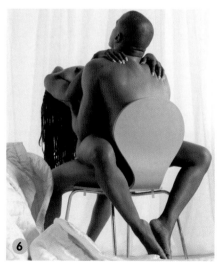

6

7 Skin-on-skin contact

This "spoons" position is considered to be the least active of the sexual positions. It is perfect to do first thing in the morning when you just want some meditative and relaxing sex, on a lazy, hot afternoon or late at night when you're feeling romantic but sleepy. It is wonderfully cosy and very intimate, with lots of cuddling and caressing. It is good for tired people and those who aren't very agile or if you are pregnant.

When you are lying down with your back to your partner, curl your knees up and snuggle your bottom towards him. This is pure skin-on-skin contact. If he has only a partial erection, place his penis between your thighs and squeeze them together. Once he is up to speed, you can guide him into you – lean forwards if the angle is too shallow.

At the same time, reach back and massage his testicles or slowly masturbate him in between penetration sessions. You can also suck or nibble at his fingers. By lifting your leg over his, you can massage his thigh with the inner surface of yours – a surprisingly sensual sensation.

This position is great for a first-thing wake-up call, as stale morning breath can be avoided. It also gives him the chance to whisper sexy things in your ear.

8 The cross

To spice things up a little from the basic spoons position, interlock your legs, then lean forwards, while he leans back. Keeping his penis inside you as you move can take a few goes, and quite a few laughs, to get right, so hold on tight. Once you have managed this stage, with some careful choreography you should be able to keep swivelling your bodies, so that both heads end up between each other's legs. Grab each other's hands or shoulders to prevent yourselves coming apart. This position requires both verbal and non-verbal communication and co-ordination, and slow movements.

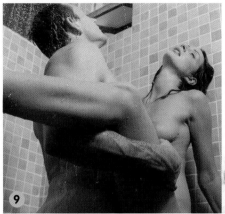

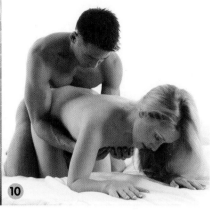

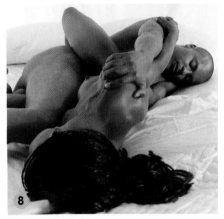

9 Shower head

This is one you see regularly in movies, whether it's in the shower, up against a garden wall, or against a door. It's fantastic for passionate, spur-of-the-moment sex in a place where you never expected it to happen. Standing positions are very exciting, although penetration is not deep.

Don't wait for him to suggest it. If you're both in the shower, lather up your hands with soap and wash him all over, leaving the pubic area until last, but then rinse this area thoroughly, as soap may sting if used for lubrication. Use the wall for balance, or, if the shower cubicle looks a bit shaky, you

will have to lean on him. With one arm around his neck, you can massage all down his spine and buttocks with the other.

Once he has got the idea, you can proceed. If you are athletic, you can fling a leg over his shoulder. The rest of us will have to be content with wrapping a leg around his waist. If he holds your leg for you, all the better: it will hold you steady while he thrusts.

Of course, you could always nuzzle your behind up to him suggestively and let him take you from the rear. Entry from behind is fantastic for deep, penetrative sex. The penis is naturally angled to maximize impact for clitoral stimulation, although you may still need a little manual assistance, and the man's testicles rub and bounce against the vulva with each stroke, creating a most sensuous feeling for both partners. You don't have to be in a shower, of course: up against a full-length mirror is sexy, too; in fact, this is a great position for being partially clothed almost anywhere.

10 From behind

This a position that brings out the primal urges in many men. It is going to be difficult to instigate this one, as he needs to take control – but that doesn't mean you can't take the initiative. If you are on all fours, present your behind to him, and he probably

will not need to be asked twice. If you can, lean back and stroke his testicles to encourage him.

This is a difficult angle for penetration, so he might need some assistance. It is helpful to have something to lean forwards on, be it a table, bed, wall or chair. When your arms get tired, you will probably end up with your head on the bed, but you need to keep your bottom lifted in the air to keep the correct angle for penetration. Hook your legs around him so you can have some control, as he is guaranteed to be pumping by now. From here, you can straighten your legs and arms, and make like a wheelbarrow. You can try this where you are lying face down on the bed with your legs over the edge, so he can hold them while he is standing or kneeling down.

This is great for an intense passionate romp, as both partners are aroused very quickly. If he kneels up, the man can see his penis moving in and out, and he also has a tantalizing view of his partner's body. Lots of laughs are guaranteed. This is great when you are in a really raunchy mood and want to feel like porn stars. Perfecting the technique is fairly tricky, but enormous fun. This isn't a position for the long haul embrace, as the blood will run to your head, but he will love you for suggesting it.

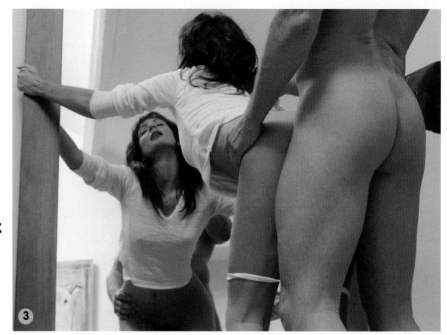

10 top places for great sex

It is not just sexual positions that can spice up sex, but where you have sex as well – men particularly can get a thrill from a change of scene. Do remember that having sex in public places is a criminal offence. With a bit of imagination, however, most of these can be re-created in the privacy of your own home (or garage for the vehicular variety). Just having sex in the hallway makes a change, and you'll never be able to pass that hall mirror again without smiling quietly to yourself. Why not make it your aim to make love at least once in every room of the house? And don't forget the garden, then there's the loft, the shed….

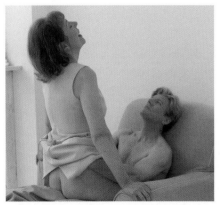

1 The beach
This is going to be no fun in the middle of the day on a crowded bathing beach. So wait until everyone has taken their towels and children home for the day, and the moon is shining romantically in the sky. Choose your spot carefully – sand dunes are good for providing privacy, though you'll need to watch out for sand in your underwear. If it's a pebble beach, whoever is underneath will get a good massage, or bruises, into the bargain. Perhaps this is a good time for you to suggest going on top.

2 Lovers' lane
Wherever you live, there will be lonely lanes where lovers have traditionally gone to have sex away from the watchful eyes of their parents (or partners). This is the old 1950s cliché, with the rocking car and the steamed-up windows. It might not be so much fun in the back of your nippy hatchback, but where there's a will, there's a way.

3 In front of a mirror
You'll be amazed at how the presence of a mirror – preferably a giant one – can turn good sex into something much more erotic. Rear entry is best here, so that you can both watch yourselves starring in your own private porn show, and he gets to see you from the front and back at the same time. Watching yourself orgasm is the icing on the cake.

4 An elevator
Remember to press "stop" first – otherwise you will have to be really quick to accomplish this one. For those of you who have watched too many thriller movies, it might be a little daunting. You have to try to forget all that safety advice about how to survive a plunging elevator. And jumping in the air when he is about to climax will not be a popular move. When you get out, you may see some amused security men – don't wait until afterwards to notice the closed-circuit television cameras.

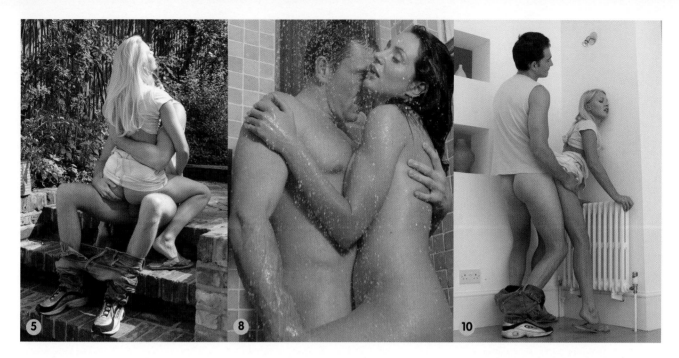

5 Al fresco

Sex can be just as thrilling in your own garden as in some secluded field: the risk of being seen adds a certain frisson to the occasion. Add to that the feeling of the sun on your bodies, and fresh air in all sorts of interesting places, and you're on to a winner.

6 Underwater loving

If you've rocked the boat and gone overboard, you may as well make the most of the underwater environment. Many people like the idea of having sex in water, but have heard horror stories about couples getting stuck together after a steamy session in the swimming pool. This is exceedingly rare and only possible if the right combination of vaginal contraction and force of suction is applied. A more realistic concern is that of infection, especially if the aquatic lovemaking takes place in a public area, such as a swimming pool, or a natural environment, such as a lake or stream. Having sex in

water causes water to be pumped into the vagina, and there is a possibility that micro-organisms or impurities in the water could cause irritation or infection when introduced to your internal environment. Water is, however, a very erotic element, and kissing, cuddling, fondling and foreplay are all safe aqueous activities.

7 Join the mile high club

This is the stuff of sexy novellas: nipping from your seats in economy class to have sex squashed up against the toilet rolls in a tiny airplane cubicle. However, these days there are actually some airlines that cater for copulating couples, with special beds supplied for the purpose.

8 The shower

No, not like the shower scene from *Psycho*. This is a gentler, erotic shower, with plenty of hot water to create a steamy atmosphere. Make sure that you have a good solid

shower cubicle, or else one thrust and you will have to explain the mess to the plumber. Hot tubs and Jacuzzis are also great spots for a sexy rendezvous. Bear in mind, though, that condoms won't be much use in the water.

9 The office

Late-night office romance may lead to sex on the desk. Make sure the boss isn't there, unless it's the boss you're doing, of course. If you are indulging in some intimate late-night photocopying, make sure you clean up the evidence before the next day.

10 A roadside motel

For a spontaneous afternoon of passion, book in as Mr and Mrs Smith, whether you are married or not – it's bound to raise an eyebrow from the receptionist. There is nothing like an anonymous environment to spice up your reactions to each other: you may not even make it as far as the bed.

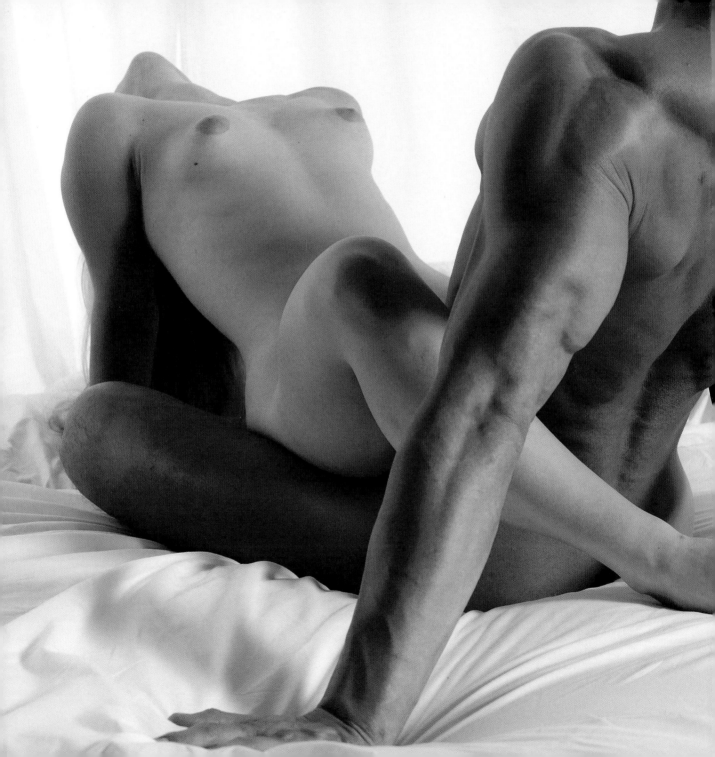

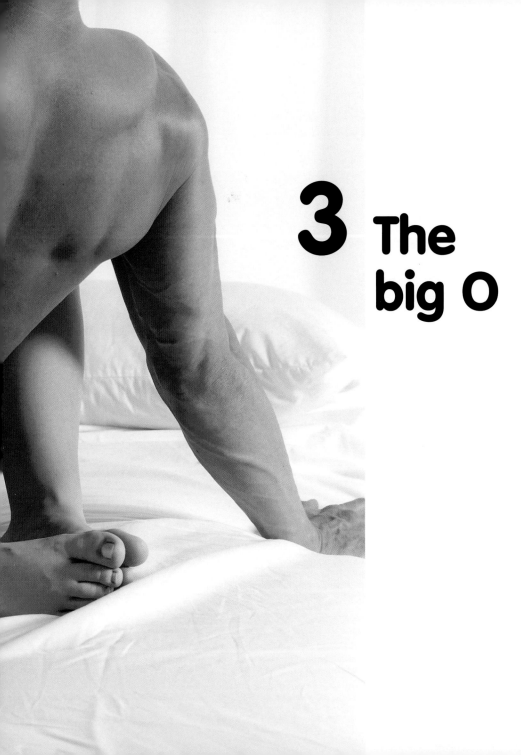

3 The big O

…relaxed, energized or exhausted, ecstatic, overjoyed or tearful, but always absolutely wonderful…

Orgasm

The climax, the goal – the pressure is on to achieve the biggest and best orgasms. Orgasms last seconds or minutes. They trigger divine sensations throughout the body, starting in the pelvis and genital area and sending overwhelming waves of delight rushing through you. They can make you feel relaxed, energized or exhausted, ecstatic, overjoyed or tearful, but always absolutely wonderful – and the even better news is that they are also good for you.

For a man, orgasm is a relatively simple process. He becomes aroused, is stimulated to the point of no return and ejaculates, although there are techniques, notably Tantrism, for achieving orgasm without ejaculation. For women, orgasm has always been more controversial and complicated.

Here, we are concerned with how you can make orgasms a more intense experience for your man, and how to ensure you have them too. For both sexes there is performance anxiety, and a certain amount of faking goes on – go on, admit it – to make the partner feel better.

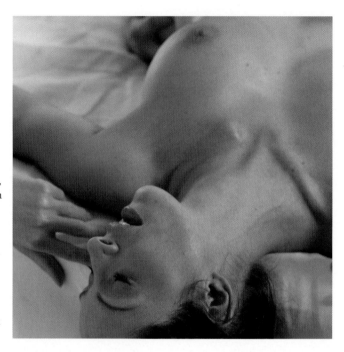

What women need to know about male orgasms

When a man becomes aroused, his penis stiffens, his heart rate increases and his muscles tighten. The most obvious signs of the build-up towards orgasm are in the penis and testicles: the veins start to bulge, the colour of the glans (head) becomes darker and the testicles rise up towards the body. Once the penis is standing at its biggest, the ridge around the head becomes extra sensitive and the man has reached the point of no return. He will then orgasm, in up to eight contractions, at around one-second intervals.

The blissful sensations of orgasm come, in part, from the seminal fluid exploding into the urinary passage deep in the prostate gland. Most men experience orgasm as sensation and ejaculation, but some men have experienced whole-body orgasms, usually by delaying ejaculation through will or by using Tantric techniques. This mind-over-matter approach may not work for other problems, however. Reaching orgasm may just take time if he is over-anxious about making everything work out well, or if he has something else on his mind. Anxiety often plays a major causal role for men in premature ejaculation. This is also true of repeated failure to maintain an erection. However, more often than not, both these problems are occasional and can be resolved with patience, understanding and a little imagination on your part. There may be a physical cause, so get him to check with his doctor if the problem persists.

The aftermath is called the refractory period, during which the body recovers from the orgasm. This can take anything from a few minutes to several days, depending on age (his, not yours).

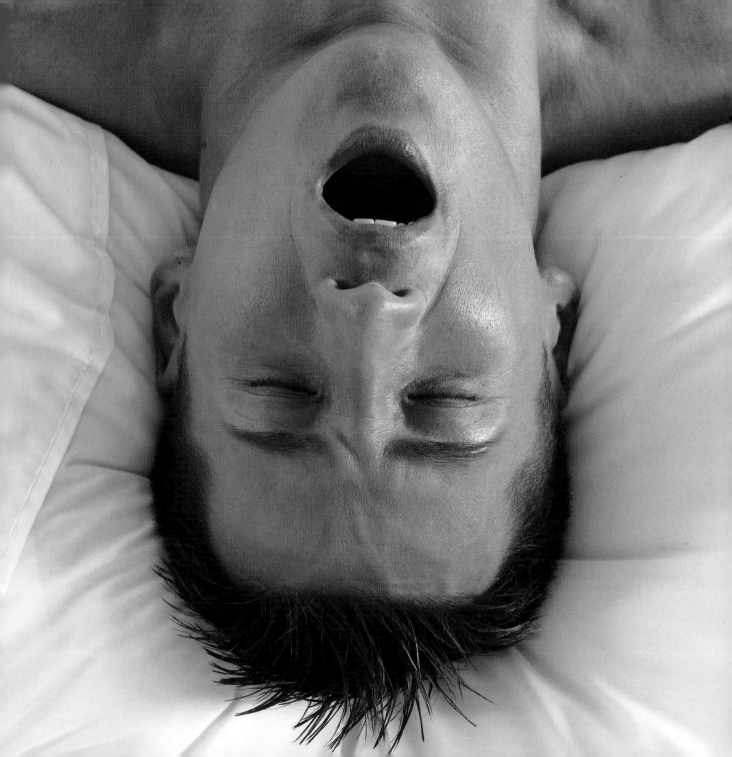

10 tips for the ultimate orgasm

An orgasm will unleash different sensations according to the different methods used to reach it: masturbation, oral sex or penetration. It is often said that orgasm through masturbation, for example, is more intense than orgasm with a partner, because we ourselves know the best means of delivery. There is no one way of having the ultimate orgasm. Some men need only look at a naked woman; while others will need copious amounts of encouragement from you. Everyone is different, and you must explore the options to find which methods are most satisfying for both of you.

Some men say that having their testicles stroked at orgasm heightens the sensation; others love it when their nipples are sucked. The nearest a man will ever get to a multiple orgasm, though, will probably be when he's a teenager and can ejaculate several times in a row. If a man has a second orgasm within a couple of hours, the sensations can be much more intense. There is no proven medical explanation for this, but one reason may be that his senses have been heightened by his first orgasm.

Of course, you need to make sure that you are having your fair quota of orgasms, and these tips should help you do along the way.

1 Simultaneous orgasm

This is said to be the ultimate goal of lovemaking. If it happens, then climaxing at the same time is fantastic. However, not many couples manage it, so don't be too disappointed if you aren't among the lucky few. In fact, there are reasons why it may not be such a good idea. What about watching your partner orgasm? Isn't that the most erotic thing in the world? And if you are concentrating on your own orgasm, there can be a sense of dislocation in which you feel momentarily separated from him at the most important moment.

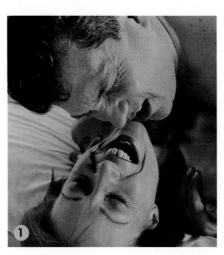

2 The pelvic floor

Getting your pelvic floor muscles in shape will not only help your queenly milking, (see point 3) but will also increase your own responses, as it is the same muscles which support the clitoris. If you haven't located these yet, try to stop the flow of urine next time you are on the toilet. Those are the ones you want to exercise, several times a day. Once you have found the muscles, try contracting them gradually, in small stages, releasing them in the same controlled way. You'll begin to feel an improvement in no time – and so will he.

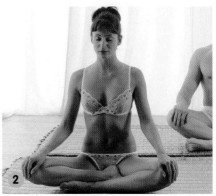

3 The G spot

The male G spot is his prostate gland which, when stimulated, can produce the most wonderful orgasms, sometimes even if his penis isn't being touched. The nerve pathway from the penis to the brain runs through the rectum and a nerve centre is located beneath the prostate, so the sensations are powerful and intense. A lubricated finger inserted into his anus – avoid long fingernails – will find the walnut-sized prostate gland about 5cm/2in up, towards the navel.

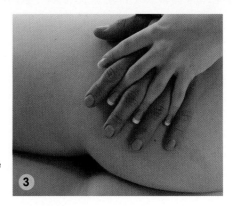

4 Cleopatra's kiss

The Egyptian queen Cleopatra must have known a thing or two about keeping her men folk happy in the sack. "Cleopatra's kiss" is the name given to the rhythmic squeezing of the vaginal muscles, also known as "milking". The sensation is guaranteed to drive him wild. Some positions make this easier to practise than others. Often being on top is the best, but experiment to see what works for you.

5 The rising towel

His performance will also be improved if you can persuade him to exercise his pelvic floor. He can do the same exercise as you, or you can try balancing a piece of kitchen paper on his erect penis. Ask him to contract his pelvic floor muscles, so that the towel moves up and down. The longer he can hold the contraction, the stronger the muscles become.

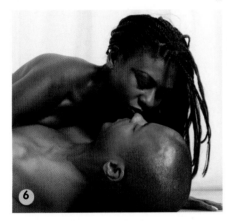

6 Stop and start

For men, extended sexual pleasure has to be mastered. The longer that foreplay continues, the more intense the orgasm. To make his experience one that he won't forget, keep him on a short rein. Just when you feel he may be reaching the point of no return, stop what you are doing. Slow down your movements so that he returns, momentarily, from the brink. Then start up again, taking him back to the edge, before stopping again. This might drive him mad with frustration to start with, but when he achieves the hottest orgasm he's ever had, he'll be sure to thank you.

7 Rock and roll

If your partner sees that you are really enjoying yourself, that will turn him on more than any fancy moves. Genuinely throw yourself into the spirit of the occasion: scream, wriggle, and generally squirm about so he can tell you are still there. Lying still and keeping quiet isn't very encouraging. When he thrusts his pelvis, thrust back and try to catch the rhythm so you are both going in the same direction. There's a good reason why it is called the bump and grind.

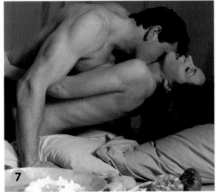

8 The squeeze

You may have a man who goes in for Tantra classes, or has pelvic floor muscles of steel, but if not you can try the squeeze technique. Just before orgasm, place your thumb on one side of the base of the penis and the tips of your index and middle fingers on the other side, then squeeze. This stops the blood flow to the penis, slowing everything down, and giving you time to catch up.

9 Faking it

It's not only women who fake orgasms. Many men do it too, probably because of the same kind of insecurities from which women suffer. If your man fails to orgasm, it is not a good idea to insist that you help him have one – just let it be for a little while. Pursuing the issue may make things worse.

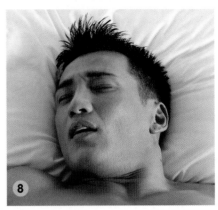

10 Spectator sport

Broaching the subject of masturbating in front of each other can be tricky, but the benefits can be well worth it. Many couples enjoy mutual masturbation as a safer means of enjoying each other without penetration. Masturbation can result in some of the most intense orgasms, and it seems only reasonable that these experiences should be witnessed. Most people will jump at the chance of watching their loved one having a great time and sharing the pleasure. Take the opportunity of watching your partner to observe how he likes to be touched. Try laying your hand over his as he stimulates himself. That way you will become attuned to the rhythm he likes best.

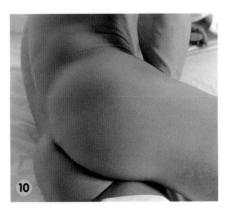

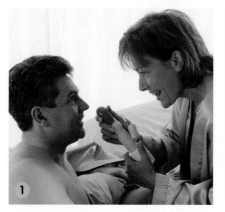

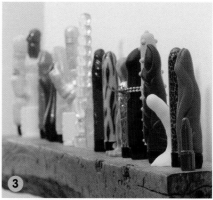

10 hot toys and how to use them...

Sex toys are coming out of the bedside drawer and going on the coffee table – and they're not just for women. There are as many gizmos and gadgets for men, from anal love balls to penis rings, as there are for women. We are becoming more open to the idea of incorporating toys into sex play and less bashful about enjoying them.

The whole purpose of sex toys is fun, but you may need to be careful about how you introduce the idea to your partner. Many men feel that they are being criticized as inadequate lovers if their partner buys a vibrator. Reassure your partner that you don't prefer the toys to him – it's just a different and fun variation: sometimes you like oral sex, sometimes penetration and sometimes playing with toys.

People have been using sex toys since time immemorial. Wooden and china love balls, for example, were used in ancient China. Remember, though, that you should always use toys designed for the purpose, rather than improvising. Emergency doctors can produce the most horrific lists of items that have got lost inside a vagina or anus at some time. This is actually very dangerous – the only amusing thing being the excuses people give for the presence of the objects.

1 Shopping spree

Why not buy him a toy as a present? It will be obvious then that you intend it for his use, not that he is being put out of a job. Or you could go on a shopping expedition together. Chances are neither of you has been into a sex shop before, and the experience itself may prove to be as thrilling as anything you can buy – there is a whole new generation of erotic emporia to cater for modern couples.

2 Erogenous ecstasy

Sex toys are great incorporated into foreplay. A small, flexible vibrator with rubber nodules is just as great for stimulating his G-spot as it is for stimulating yourself. Most vibrators are good for external stimulation as well as penetration, and will feel fabulous on his erogenous zones, such as the insides of his thighs. Try massaging his perineum and testicles: that should give him a buzz.

3 Good vibrations

It's easy to confuse a vibrator with a dildo, so what is the difference? Well, the vibrator vibrates and the dildo doesn't. Although generally thought of as the preserve of women going solo, vibrators can also be used by men to stimulate their penises. They can, of course, also be used by men to bring women to orgasm, and vice versa.

4 Battery power

Experiment with the different sensations a vibrating toy can produce. It can be used for massaging the clitoris, penis, testicles or anus. Try holding one between you while you are having sex, so that it comes into contact with your clitoris and his testicles, then you will both feel the benefit.

Always wash and dry your toys after use, and remember to keep a supply of batteries handy, as there are few things worse than a pre-orgasmic power failure.

5 Anal beads

If you really want to surprise your man with something new, a set of anal beads should do the trick. As their name suggests, these are a string of beads, often gradating in size, designed to be inserted in his back passage. Men report fabulous sensations when they are pulled out quickly at the moment of climax. Perhaps the contractions of the anus add to the fun, or the friction of the beads running over his G-spot. Whatever the reason, it might be worth a try, but don't forget to use plenty of lubrication and to leave at least part of the toy outside the body.

6 Cock rings

These little devices might be some of the oldest sex toys around, and are certainly a small and discreet gift for him. The idea is

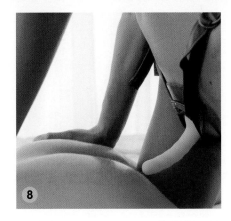

8

that a ring is placed around an erect penis, where it constricts the blood flow, thus helping to maintain the erection for longer. An added bonus is the sensations you will feel during penetration, but then it was never intended as a totally selfless present, was it?

7 Dildos

Dildos are usually phallic in shape, and have a history that stretches back 30,000 years, so if you're feeling embarrassed about buying one, remember you are by no means the first. Regular use of a dildo can help to strengthen the vaginal walls by exercising the muscles. When buying a dildo intended for anal penetration, make sure that it has a flared end so it can't disappear up the rectum. This may save you an embarrassing emergency trip to the local hospital.

8 Harness your power

Used in conjunction with dildos for strap-on sex, harnesses allow the wearer to ignore gender boundaries, so that you can anally penetrate your partner or he can penetrate your vagina and your anus at the same time. A strap-on lets you know what it feels like to be the penetrator, rather than the penetratee. Its use enables couples to role-play, and has unlimited possibilities. Just the sight of you wearing it could be all the stimulation he needs.

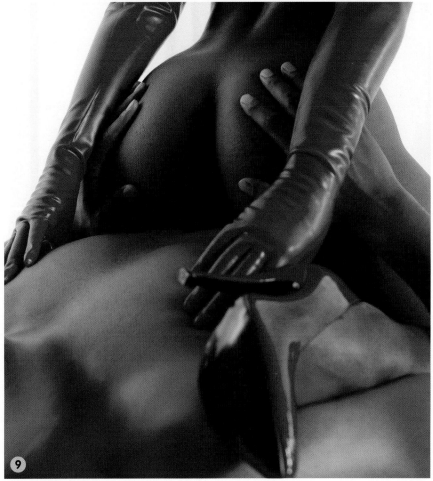

9

9 Sensation seekers

Some men are attracted by tactile adventures. Try some satin evening gloves to raise the tone – even those woolly gloves your granny gave you last Christmas might have the same effect. Rubber gloves can work well – you must just hope he has a sense of humour when he sees your pink household mitts. You can buy gloves specially made with different fabrics on each finger for a handful of fun. While you are at it, why not try on some matching heels? It's sure to create a sensation.

10 Lubrication

There is nothing worse than having to stop a steamy session because of drying up, so always keep some lubrication handy. The production of love juice is not necessarily directly related to how aroused you both are – in fact, it is hormone-controlled.

Lubrication is an essential component in anal play, as the anus and surrounding area produce no natural lubrication. Be sure to use water-based lubricants if you are using condoms, so as not to damage them.

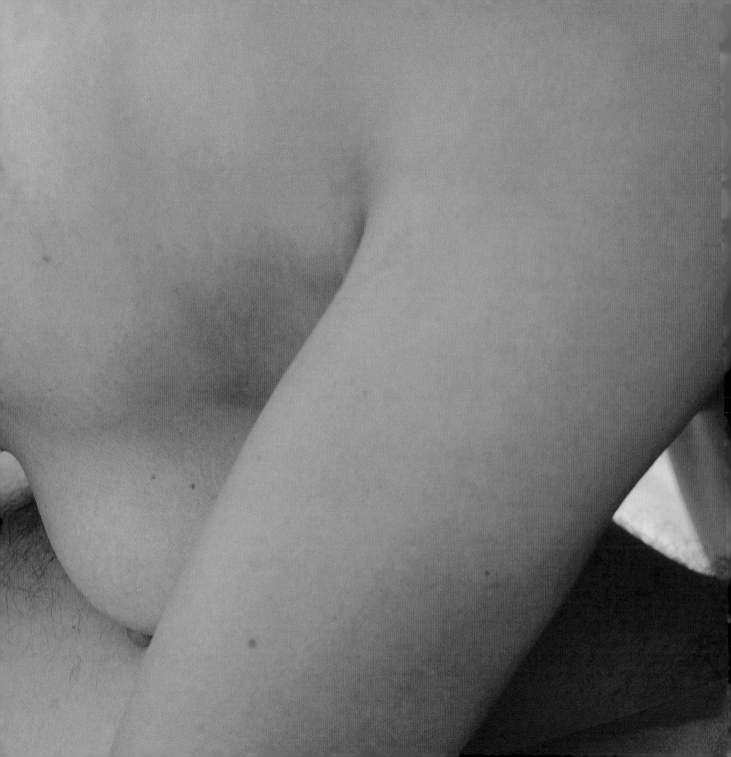

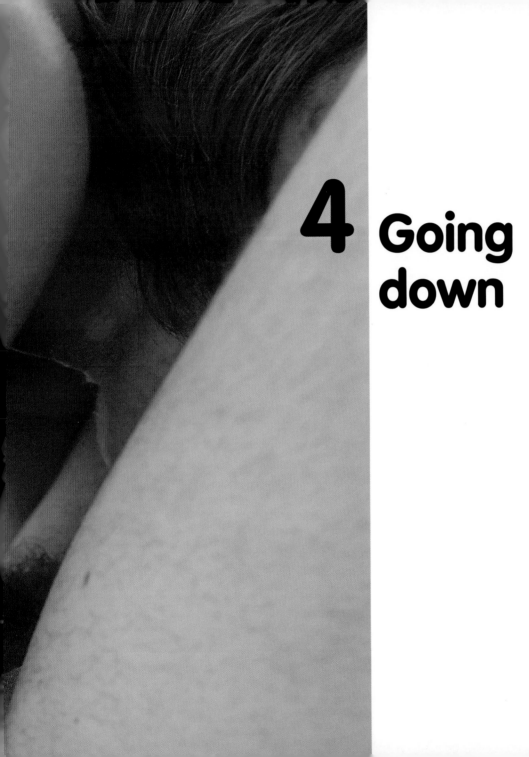

4 Going down

…Listen to your partner's moans and watch his body movements to work out what is working for him and what isn't…

What every woman should know about oral sex

The art of oral sexuality has been greatly neglected. Most men are rather keen, while the majority of women have some ambivalence. Oral sex is a major part of lovemaking and is not to be dismissed lightly. Frank discussion with your man is obviously a starting point to breaking down any barriers that may exist. Knowledge can be the next step, as forewarned is forearmed.

For many women, oral sex is a sure route to orgasm, so if you want him to go down on you, it's only fair to reciprocate, isn't it? And, after all, there is nothing more sensual and pleasurable than lying back and letting the cares of the world pass you by. Too many people think of oral sex as a prelude to penetrative sex. In fact, it is a quite separate act. The techniques used for explosive oral sex are extremely different from those of penetrative sex. By refining the art, you can get a greater understanding of your partner's sexual preferences. It is an exciting journey of exploration into your partner's hot spots – a journey that will be even more exciting for him.

Talking and timing

In order to be an oral aficionado, the secret is a combination of timing, listening and responding. Once again, it's all to do with communication. Take time with oral sex, and do it sometimes just for its own sake. Listen to your partner's moans and watch his body movements to work out what is working for him and what isn't. Respond according to what is working, and keep doing it.

Make it apparent to your partner that you are enjoying yourself too. Oral sex is not something you just do to someone else: you are participating and sharing in the activity and relishing the intimacy, the effects you are having and, in fact, the entire experience. (If you're not really enjoying it, perhaps you shouldn't be doing it at all.)

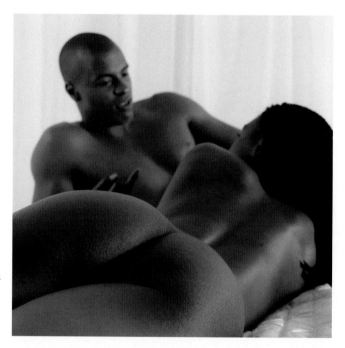

Putting your mouth around a man's penis requires trust on both sides. You assume that he has washed his penis and that he won't choke you by thrusting in too far, and he assumes that no biting will be involved – something men commonly have nightmares about. Some women have been put off by a man holding their head down to restrict their movements. Make him understand that unless he accepts that this is a no-no you will not proceed.

The secret to giving good head is, without a doubt, enthusiasm rather than technique. The mere idea of a blow-job is a massive turn-on for him. If you don't want to do it, then simply refrain – a half-hearted effort will disappoint him and make you resentful. If you are willing to give it a try, then arm yourself with the hot tips here, and take it slowly, one step at a time.

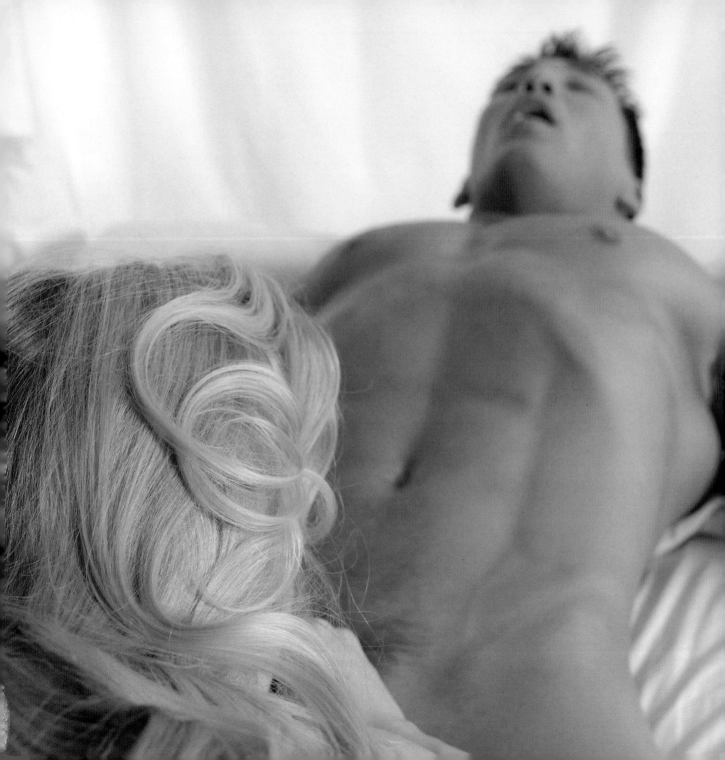

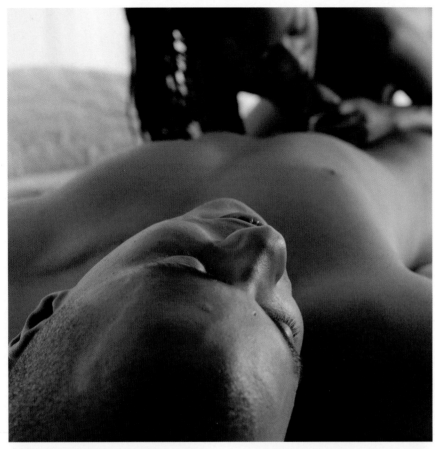

10 hot tips for fantastic fellatio

The best blow-jobs are those given as a luxurious, time-consuming package. Rather than heading straight for the penis, it's often more exciting to incorporate an element of anticipation. So don't go straight for your target, but amble your way, tantalizingly, via a circuitous route.

Don't panic – unless you are very experienced, you are not going to get the whole of his member in your mouth, so don't even try. The most sensitive part of the penis is the tip anyway, so you can just use your lips and tongue to stimulate this part, without going any farther. Give it a go, and if you are not sure, let your hands take over until you have decided whether to go back down, or not.

The term "blow-job" is a misnomer, as you don't actually need to blow. As you go up and down the penis, you can create an airtight seal with your lips. This means that as you move up the penis, a vacuum will naturally create suction, so you don't have to. Use quite a firm grip with your mouth, and twist your head around at the same time for added stimulation. Use your tongue too, applying extra pressure or using a quick flicking action. He won't know what's hit him.

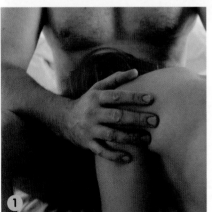

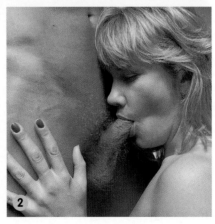

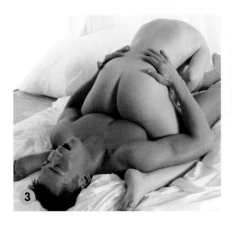

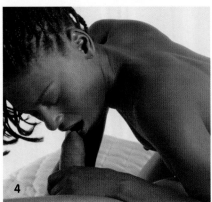

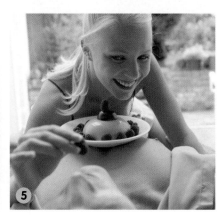

1 Take your time

Lie him flat on his back and begin either at his feet, working up, or at his chest, working down. The secret here is to ignore time and to immerse yourself in both his body and his needs, and to concentrate. Sucking toes, licking nipples, massaging his inner thighs and flicking a tongue around his navel are just some of the delights you can provide for him, but stay away from the genital area to begin with. He will see the road you are on, so as you start to home in towards his groin, he will be bursting with excitement. Once down there, you can tease him by licking around the outline of his penis on his belly, allowing your breath to pass over it, or brushing your lips suggestively over the head of his penis before using direct stimulation.

2 Lip service

Lubrication will make the process easier, so make sure you have a wet mouth and keep a drink handy. If you are not going to take him completely in your mouth, use a lot of saliva to lubricate the lower part of the shaft, which you can stimulate with your hands. Wrap your lips over your teeth – the merest hint of anything sharp near a man's penis will have him leaping away from you in fear. You are simulating penetration, but you will have much better control over your lips and hands than you do over your vaginal muscles.

3 Flexible friend

Get your tongue working. Little flicks of the tongue around the head and over the frenulum are very stimulating and will make your partner think he's in heaven. Roll your tongue both quickly and slowly around the head, stimulating both the frenulum and the glans. This is sure to get him going if he is not stiff yet. Just hold the base of his penis and squeeze it firmly while your tongue does its magical work.

4 Combined effort

A good blow-job is a partnership of both the mouth and the hands. While your mouth concentrates mainly on the top end of his penis, your hands can be working on the lower shaft. The most successful technique is to synchronize your movements, allowing your hands to follow the pumping action of your mouth. Use either one or two hands to follow your mouth up and down the shaft, gripping it as you would a tennis racket. You can have quite a firm grip – the firmer the better, as far as he is concerned. If you sit on him facing his feet, he gets to stroke (and look at) your bottom while you're in action.

The head of the penis is often more sensitive in uncircumcised men. You can place the tip of your tongue underneath the foreskin and run circles around the head, or you can pull the foreskin back with your

hands by wrapping them around the shaft, just above the base, and pulling down to the base. This exposure heightens sensitivity and will make it more exciting for him.

Another technique worth trying is called "flicking". During a blow-job, slide the shaft out of your mouth and then flick his penis gently against your cheek or neck a few times; you get a breather, and he gets a different sensation.

5 Spicing it up

Experimentation with different tastes and textures can spice up a blow-job even more. Try sucking on a mint beforehand: the added ingredient of menthol in your saliva will provide a different sensation on your partner's penis. Don't be tempted to use anything too strong directly on his skin, or it won't just be a tingle he feels, and you could cause some damage to his sensitive skin. Sucking ice cubes or licking ice cream and then drinking hot drinks also adds variety. Your favourite spreads, such as chocolate or jam, can also make it a tastier experience for you, and you can have lots of fun with the application.

What he has eaten can make a difference to how his sperm tastes. Any asparagus recently, and your taste buds will certainly know about it. Some people claim vanilla ice cream has a pleasant effect on the taste.

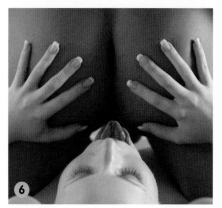

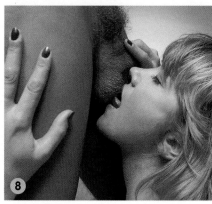

6 Rimming

Some men like to have their prostate or anus stimulated during oral sex, and many of them say that orgasm is greatly heightened when the prostate is stimulated at the same time. Using a little lubrication, massage around the area for a while to relax him before gradually slipping in one finger. Once inside, very gently massage the area towards his navel, taking care not to scratch with your fingernail.

Licking or probing the anus with the tongue, known as analingus or rimming, is also a source of pleasure for some men. This is a good way to explore the idea of anal penetration, as the mouth supplies all the lubrication you need. For some men this is a slightly forbidden thrill, but others may interpret any play with the back passage as a questioning of their masculinity, so tread carefully on this issue.

7 Variations on a theme

From this point there are a variety of techniques that you can use. Different men like to be stimulated in different ways, so why not try them all and see which ones he likes the most? You can discuss what his likes and dislikes are, or simply read his body. If he's groaning and grinding, then you are on to a winner. If he is quieter or pulling away from you, try something else.

First of all, position yourself so that you are comfortable. Most women like to be between their partner's legs, with him lying back. This positions the tongue so that it can easily stimulate the front of the penis, the most sensitive area, and also allows your partner to look down and watch you in action, which will excite him even more.

Hold his penis in one hand and place your lips at the bottom end of the shaft on the top side. Use your lips as if you were kissing, and create a light suction, then move your mouth and head steadily up and down the shaft, increasing and decreasing the pace. You can use your other hand to caress the head or glans of his penis at the same time.

"Rolling" produces a wonderful sensation, as it concentrates on the head of the penis, the most sensitive area. Place your mouth over the head of the penis so that it is completely in your mouth. Use your tongue to stroke all around the edges of the head in a circular motion, quickening and lessening the pace and changing direction every now and again. When your tongue passes over the frenulum at the front of the head (facing you), use the bit of skin that attaches your tongue to the bottom of your mouth to stimulate it. You can also use your tongue to massage the tip, as if you were licking an ice cream (it's true, ice cream really is sexy).

8 Ball games

Men's testicles are very sensitive, and you can give a lot of pleasure by playing with them. Just before a man comes, his balls contract and move up towards his body to prepare for ejaculation. By gently gripping them at the top and pulling them down (gently, gently), you can hold off his orgasm. Put his balls in your mouth, sucking and licking them – massaging them with your tongue can produce a wonderful sensation.

There are many ways to alter the sensations he will feel, so experiment until you find something that he goes crazy for. As you are sucking him, try humming, singing or moaning at the same time, as the vibrations from your voice box will penetrate through to his penis and make it more stimulating. You could also try holding a string of pearls (any beads will do) in your hands as you are stroking him. The contrast of the cool beads and your hot wet mouth is sure to get his interest, and the other kind of pearl necklace might follow.

9 The swallow debate

The pros and cons of swallowing semen are individual to each woman. Some women don't like the idea of it, others wouldn't consider spitting, and see swallowing as the ultimate finale. Men's preferences on the matter vary too.

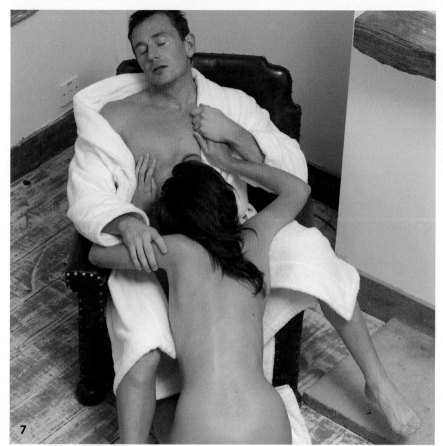

7

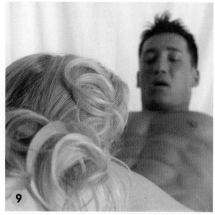

9

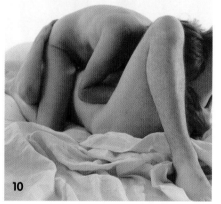

10

Knowing when a man is about to ejaculate can be quite tricky. Things to look for – apart from an obvious screaming announcement – are a tightening of the muscles and increased rate of breathing. His facial expression, if you can see it, is often a giveaway, too.

If you don't want to swallow, you can withdraw, and finish him off with your hand; alternatively, you can spit, but do it discreetly or it will put you both off. Another option is to ask him to come on your breasts, which is known as a pearl necklace, or on your face. Semen is, apparently, very good for the condition of your skin.

Most women worry about gagging. This is the natural reflex if the penis hits the back of your throat. You need to stay in control of the situation. Don't let him hold your head, and make sure you are free to move away. Keeping one hand on the base of his penis is a good way to keep the upper hand – and don't forget to breathe.

10 Soixante-neuf
The 69 is tricky. Many people find it hard to concentrate on stimulating as well as being simultaneously stimulated. It can be difficult for the man to hit your spot in this position, as his chin is stimulating your clitoris.

Similarly, it is the less sensitive top side of the penis that receives most stimulation. Height differences can cause problems, too, making one partner curl and the other stretch.

So why do it? Well, apart from the fact that it is a real giggle, it can also be quite effective. The sight of each other's most private places up so close can prove to be an astonishingly erotic experience. If you go on top, you'll be more in control, and you'll both be giving and receiving at the same time, though you might have trouble keeping at the same pace. It is hard to be relaxed enough to orgasm while you are concentrating on him, but then practice may prove to be the answer.

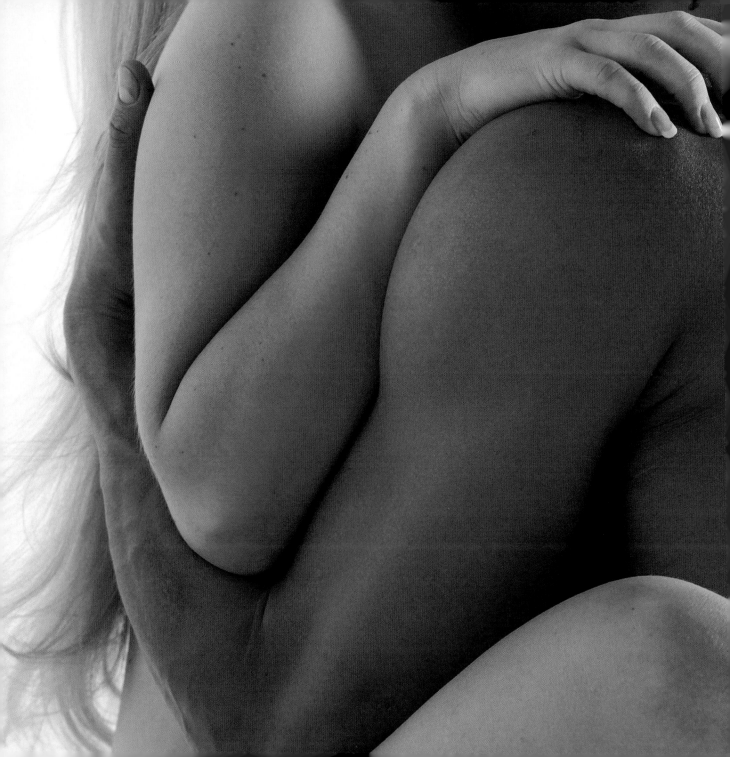

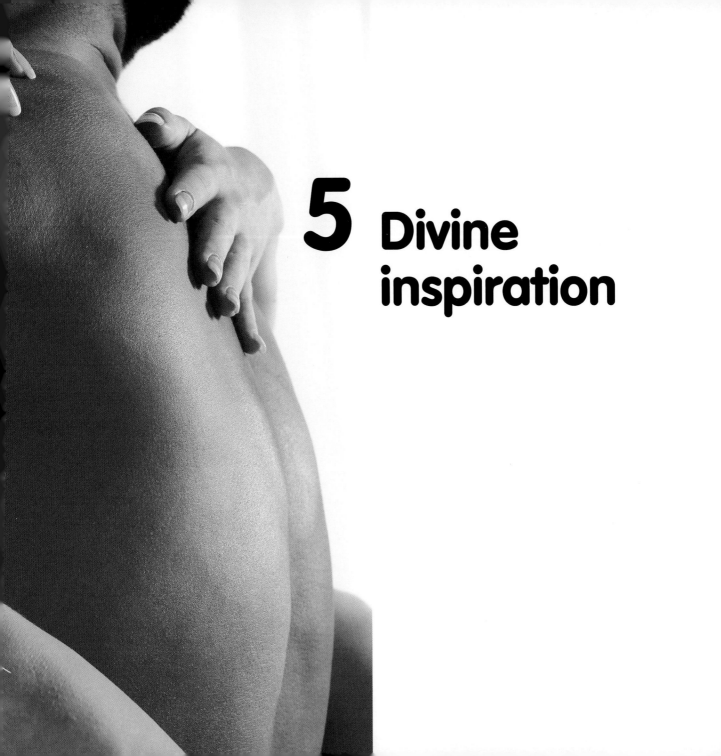

5 Divine inspiration

…there are plenty of ideas here to help you to light a fire under your man, if he is flagging…

Ancient erotica

Once you have become mistress of the basics, you'll be looking for more advanced inspiration for your lovemaking. Ancient Chinese and Indian texts have a lot to teach us, and although many of their customs differ from our own, there are essential similarities. Over the last 3,000 years, Eastern cultures have worshipped and respected the power and life force of human sexual nature. Although contemporary Western society is more liberal and open than in the past, the arts of seduction, sensuality and wanton abandon have been under-developed here by comparison. By looking towards the East, we can borrow wisdom and teachings from a long history of enlightened sexual revolutionaries.

Enlightened writings

There are several texts that have survived and been translated in the West. Most famous is the *Kama Sutra*, a Hindu text not solely sexually focused: in fact only a small portion of the text concentrates on the act of sex. It advises on other aspects of male–female relations, too, such as courtship and marriage, the duties of wife and husband, and enhancing beauty and attractiveness, and it provides a variety of recipes and incantations to help with sexual problems and difficulties. While the *Kama Sutra* does include a list of exotic positions for sex, it also describes in great detail the delicacy of foreplay and the importance of both parties being satisfied sexually, and stresses that they should share time together as a couple after congress. In India, it became a guide to human relations and interactions.

The *Ananga Ranga* written by Kalyana Malla, is a long treatise on eroticism, directed at long-term couples, with the aim of relieving "the monotony which follows possession". It incorporated the much older *Kama Sutra*, and describes a multitude of kisses, embraces and sexual positions.

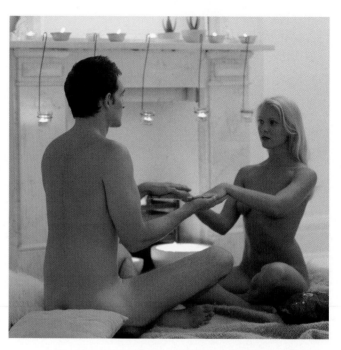

Although originally written for a male readership, the *Ananga Ranga* seeks to help couples to renew their desire for sex, which in turn helps them to re-establish strong bonds, both of friendship and love. So there are plenty of ideas here to help you to light a fire under your man, if he is flagging.

More than a practice or step-by-step guide, Tantra is a philosophy concerned with spirituality and divine energy, blending sacred sexuality, Eastern philosophy and the teachings of the *Kama Sutra*. It involves the use of meditation and yoga to master the ultimate goal of dissipating the ego and creating union with the divine energy that is within each of us. Tantra involves raising energy through the chakras and achieving kundalini, which just means, of course, bigger and better orgasms for those who practise it.

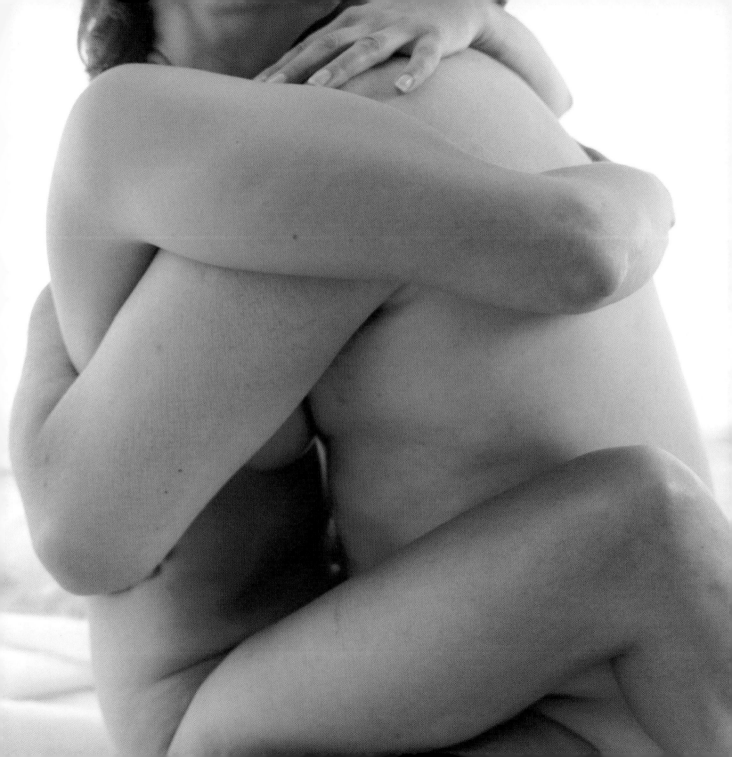

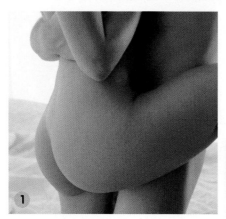

1

Tips from the Ananga Ranga

The Ananga Ranga's chapter on the "treating of external enjoyments" concentrates on the importance of various preliminaries that should precede sex, the "internal enjoyment". These include the various types of kissing and embracing, biting, scratching and hair pulling. These acts, according to Malla, "affect the senses and divert the mind from coyness and coldness".

Foreplay is an essential part of all sexual encounters, since it helps to relax and acquaint the partners with each other's bodies and erogenous zones, allowing both to reach the same levels of excitement before actual penetration.

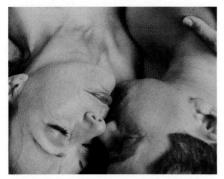

1 Embracing
As is recognized by psychosexual counsellors today, touching is one of the most mutually satisfying ways for men and women to show their affection for each other – not just when they are going to have sex, but at other times in their daily lives as well.

Vrikshadhirudha This is often referred to as the embrace that simulates climbing a tree. Place one foot on your partner's foot and raise your other leg, resting your foot upon his thigh. Put your arms around his back and hold him tightly.

Tila-tandula Stand in front of each other and hold him closely around the waist, encouraging him to do the same. Then, being careful to remain still, allow his penis to come into contact with your pubis, with only a thin veil of clothing between you. Try to stand still, although it may be hard to remain like this for a long time, as the sensation of each other's genitals in such close proximity is arousing, and, with any luck, will make him frantic with desire.

Urupaguha Stand in front of each other, then move together so that your legs are between his, with his inside thighs touching your outside thighs. This is an especially good embrace if the man is taller than you. The squeezing of your thighs provides gentle stimulation of the clitoris, and his genitals will be pressed against you, to good effect.

2 Kissing
The *Ananga Ranga* describes osculations, or kissing, as particular styles to be studied and to be practised alongside embracing. "There are seven places highly proper for osculation, in fact, where all the world kisses." These are the lower lip, both the eyes, both cheeks, the head, the mouth, the breasts and, lastly,

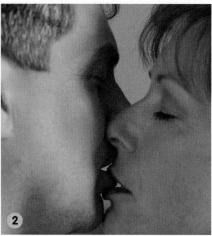

2

the shoulders. Of course there is no reason why you should stop there. Don't sit there waiting for him to make the first move – take the leading part and initiate some action.

Uttaroshtha Gently bite and nibble his lower lip, while he reciprocates on your upper lip, then swap over. This is like foreplay for kissing. You are teasing the nerve endings, so that by the time you begin a more passionate kiss, all the sensory organs in the area will be in overdrive, and aroused beyond words.

Nlita kissing When your man is angry, forcibly cover his lips with your own and continue until his anger has subsided. This type of kissing can be a fantastic means of ending an argument in which there is simply nothing more that can be said.

Ghatika kissing Cover your partner's eyes with your hands, close your own eyes and thrust your tongue into his mouth, moving it to and fro with a slow, pleasant motion that suggests another form of enjoyment. By removing one sense, in this case sight, your bodies will become more attuned to other sensations. You have turned the tables here, simulating penetration with your mouth, and therefore building anticipation about the great erotic pleasures to be indulged in later on in the proceedings.

Pratibodha When your man is sleeping, fix your lips over his, and gradually increase the pressure until sleep turns into desire. This kiss ignites passion first thing in the morning, and there is, after all, no better way to begin the day. Begin gently, then slowly become more forceful, sucking on his lips until they stir and respond.

Sphrita kissing Lean in to kiss your partner. As you approach his lower lip, jerk your mouth away without completing the kiss. A playful, teasing kiss.

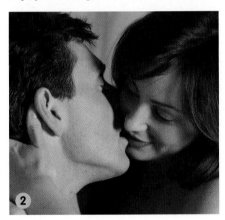

3 Scratching

The *Ananga Ranga* refers to scratching being performed as a form of remembrance, so that when you are separated there will be a mark on the body to remind you of each other. Obviously, you don't want to go making marks all over your lover, especially if he is just off to a business meeting. However, once the spark has been ignited, a little light scratching can only fan the flames. Lightly scratch your nails around his cheek, lower lip and chest. The scratching should be light enough to leave no impressions, and is more of a caress. This use of the nails, even though softly, indicates greater passion and energy than a more delicate touch.

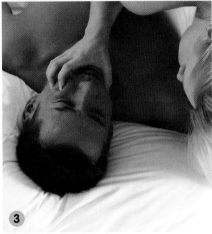

4 Biting

You won't be popular if you bite him too hard; soft nibbling is more advisable. You will have to judge timing, rising to a passionate moment with appropriate strength, and using a lighter touch when this is called for.

Uchun-dashana This is the generic term used to describe biting any part of the lips or cheeks. Gently nibbling around his face can be very sensual. Be careful around the bony areas like the cheeks, though, as they bruise easily. The lips should be handled with care, as they are protected only by a thin layer of skin, though the lower lip is very supple and elastic, and gentle sucking and nibbling on it is very pleasurable. The fleshier parts of the body, such as the thighs and buttocks, can withstand rougher treatment than the more-sensitive areas around the face.

Biting each other is a common outlet of sexual energy when in the throes of orgasm, and many people, male and female, claim that they have been surprised at the depth of a bite afterwards. Many men enjoy sharp pain at the height of passion to enhance the powerful shudders of pleasure that they experience during orgasm, but it might be a good idea to ask him first.

In the days when the *Ananga Ranga* was written, it was probably pretty acceptable for women to bear the marks of their husband's desire. Any imprint of passion on either party today, however, is reminiscent of the adolescent love bite, and not very desirable.

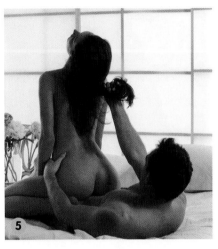

5 Hair pulling

Softly pulling the hair, states the *Ananga Ranga*, is a good method of kindling a lasting desire. Gentle pulling and playing with hair is very erotic and sensual. When pulling hair, make sure you get a good handful, as pulling at a small number of hairs can be very painful. Of course, if he doesn't have much on top, your options will be limited. Why not take it a stage further and gently pull tufts of his pubic hair – sure to bring him to a state of excitement.

It may be that he'll be more turned on by pulling your hair than having his own pulled. If you sit with your back to him, so that he can reach your hair easily, he can watch your back arch as he tugs your hair down, fantasizing about slave girls and masters.

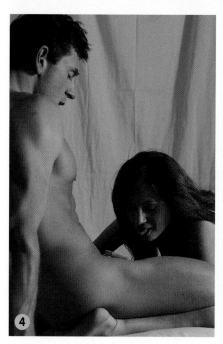

4

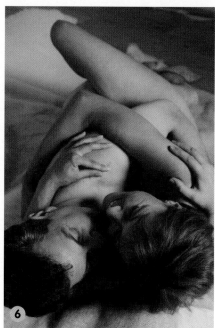

6

10 tips for exotic sex

Oral sex, known as "mouth congress" in the *Kama Sutra*, was considered a base activity practised by wanton women and eunuchs. These days it is a healthy part of most loving relationships, although some women are not sure how to go about it. Here are some more-advanced ideas for fellatio given in the *Kama Sutra* for courtesans. Knowing what you are doing will make you feel more confident, and so he will enjoy it all the more. Remember, you don't have to put the whole penis in your mouth – after all, the head is the most sensitive part.

Malla adapted many of the sexual positions in the *Ananga Ranga* from the ancient *Kama Sutra*. However, Malla's text was written in a very different social climate, where extramarital sex was frowned upon, so the emphasis is on keeping variety with one partner. Closeness continues to be important in a long-term relationship although statistics show that kissing and cuddling tend to be reduced. The Ananga Ranga sought to increase intimacy and rid marriages of any stagnation.

If you need inspiration to heat up the sheets, you will find it here. Some positions may need some participation from your partner, so leave the book open at the page you want to try, and see what happens.

1 Nimitta – touching
Holding his penis with one hand, shape your mouth into an "O" and place it on the tip of his penis. Move your head in tiny circles, maintaining a light touch.

2 Parshvatoddashta – biting to the sides
Holding the head of his penis in your hand, clamp your lips lightly above the shaft, first on one side and then the other, being careful to keep your teeth hidden.

3 Antaha-samdansha – the inner pincers
Take the whole of the head of the penis into your mouth. Press the shaft firmly between your lips, then hold it for a few seconds before pulling away.

4 Parimrshtaka – striking at the tip
Begin by flicking his penis, using a hard, pointed tongue. Then concentrate on the sensitive tip of the glans, striking it to evoke a heightened sexual sensation.

5 Sangara – swallowed whole
This is done when the man is close to orgasm. Take the whole of the penis into your mouth and suck, working with your tongue and lips until he comes.

6 Crab embrace
You may have tried this position before without realizing it. Lie on your sides facing each other. Ease one of your legs underneath his legs, and pass the other one over his body (at about the level of his navel). Help him to enter you, as it may be tricky at this angle. The position provides deep penetration and increased friction. Although his movement is limited, you will have more freedom. This is a good position if he is tired but you are feeling passionate.

7 Kama's wheel
Ask him to sit with his legs outstretched, then lower yourself on to his penis, facing him, and extend your legs. If you both

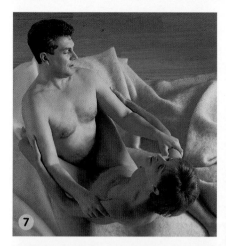

7

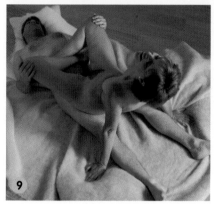

9

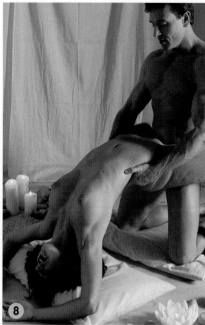

8

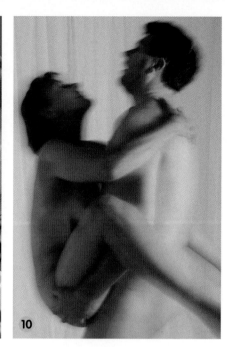

10

stretch your arms out to hold each other, this forms the wheel-like figure after which the position is named. It is said that this position combines sex and meditation to lead to a higher level of awareness. It is meant to help you both obtain a balance of mind that is clear, calm and happy.

8 Placid embrace

You will both enjoy this one, but again, you need him to help. From the Kama's wheel position, wrap your legs around his middle, lean backwards and let your head fall freely. He will have to kneel up to keep inside you, and raise you to him by grasping you around

the waist, so that your head falls towards the floor. This position allows you to retain some control – by extending and flexing the grip of your legs, you can draw him closer. Hanging with the head upside down can also contribute a feeling of ecstasy and otherworldliness for you – while for him it might just mean a work-out for his biceps.

9 Ascending position

He lies on his back while you sit cross-legged upon his thighs. Grasp his penis and insert it into yourself, moving your waist backwards and forwards as you make love to him. Since you are on top, you will be able to control the movements and depth of penetration. By moving yourself forwards and back, your clitoris also receives stimulation from the gentle rubbing action against his body. If he looks up, he gets to see all your body, and his penis going in and out. With the visual satisfaction and the increased sensation of losing control, this will drive him wild.

10 Suspended congress

You will definitely need your partner's knowing co-operation for this one. Stand opposite one another. The man bends down and passes his arms under your knees, supporting you by gripping your inner elbows or bottom. He then raises you waist high and penetrates you, while you clasp your hands around his neck to stay on.

This one could be tricky, as its success depends on factors such as the strength of the man, the weight of the woman, and the height of both. It may be easier if you get on a chair first, so that he does not have to lift you up from the ground and risk back injury. It may also help to be near a wall or rail to maintain balance. An option is to sit on the kitchen work surface, which is usually about the right height, and allows you to take some of the weight. He will love having all of you in his grasp, quite literally, and he'll be excited by having to climax before he drops you – now that would be a big bang.

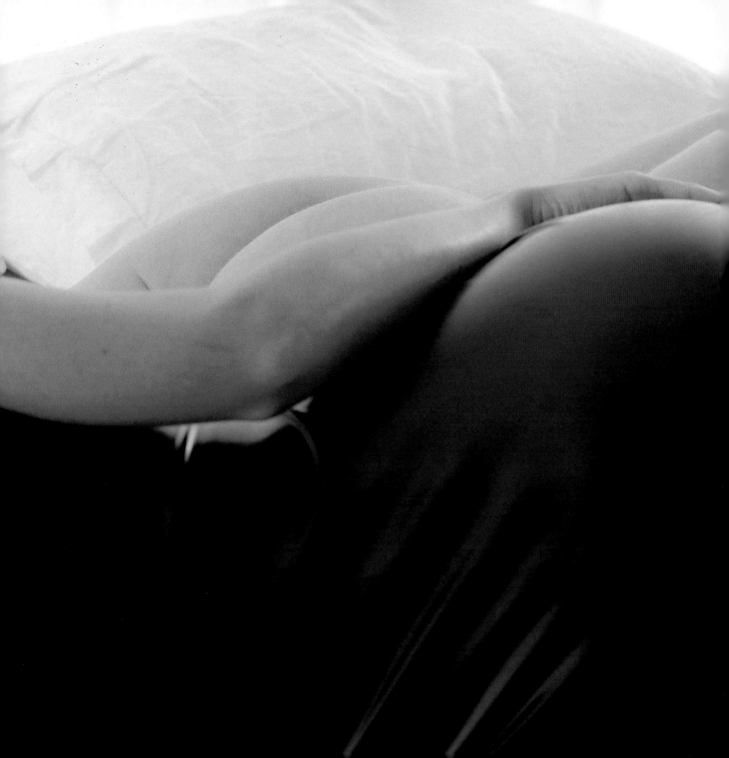

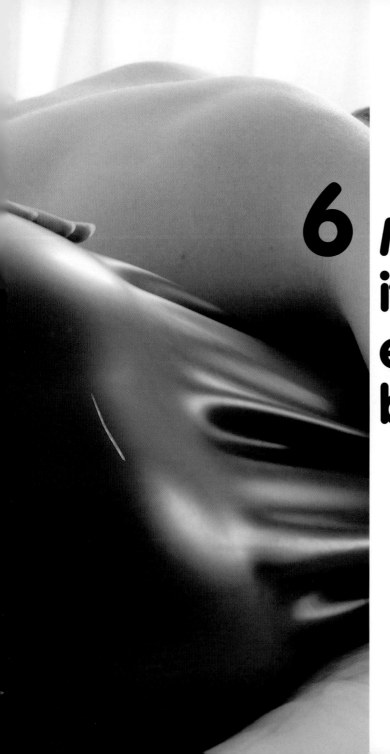

6 Making it even better

…You would think men would be tired of being dominated by women…

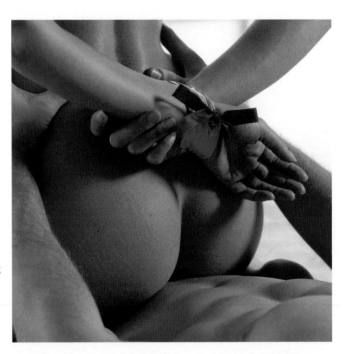

Pushing the boundaries

It is precisely because couples feel safe and comfortable together that sex can sometimes become boring. For some couples, simply letting go of a few inhibitions – and almost everyone has some – can be enough to restore the bedroom magic.

Your partner may think that trying positions and activities that haven't previously been explored could be what it takes to enliven your love life. Don't reject his suggestions out of hand; on the other hand, don't follow every idea with gritted teeth, because this leads only to resentment – on your part because you don't really want to do it and on his part because you're aren't doing it enthusiastically. If, however, your partner would like you to try, say, rimming (licking and kissing his anus) – start off by gently licking and sucking his genitals, while stroking and massaging the anal area with your hands. If you feel as though you are getting in the mood, and your partner is still keen, let your mouth follow your hands, and take it from there. If the experience makes you feel experimental yourself, get him to follow your lead – the chances are he'll want to give you the same fantastic experience you've just given him.

Acting out his fantasy

Your partner may have a desire to act out a particular fantasy. Men and women have all sorts of different ideas about what is sexy – from predictable movie-star scenarios to violent imaginings. Some men fantasize about being dominated by a woman, or several women at once. It is also know that many women fantasize about restraint, but that doesn't mean they would actually want it to happen with anyone other than their consenting partner as part of role play.

If you want to branch out, a good place to start is the Internet, as there are plenty of websites catering for all manner of sexual tastes, from swingers' clubs to voyeurism. This will give you both the

opportunity to discover the options, discuss them and form an opinion about whether you both really want to try something that, perhaps up till now, has just been a fantasy. Be prepared to indulge him in acting out his fantasies. You never know, he might then decide to return the favour...

You would think that men would be a little tired of being dominated by women, but it is still one of the most popular male fantasies. If he wants you to dress up as a dominatrix, a trip to a sex shop together would be a way to explore the possibilities. Don't get involved if you feel uncomfortable. Before you proceed with some of the more off-beat sexual thrills, set some agreed limits about what is and isn't allowed. Alternatively, you could always read raunchy magazines or books to him to indulge this aspect of his libido.

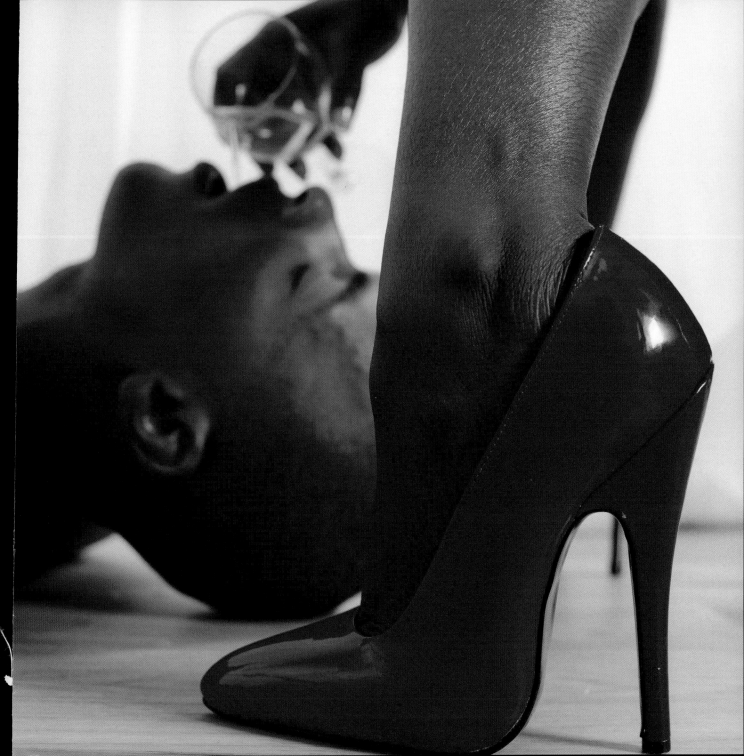

10 ways to spice it up

Doing the same old thing is going to get old, fast. You wouldn't take your boyfriend to see the same movie every week, so why use the same position every time in bed? To keep things interesting, it is important to try something new once in a while. It might not turn out to be a favourite, but hopefully you will both have had some fun in the process.

So start thinking of new possibilities, new positions, and new ways to have fun – and just make up the rules as you go along. You will end up rolling around on the carpet. And the main goal, you ask? To have a laugh and enjoy each other.

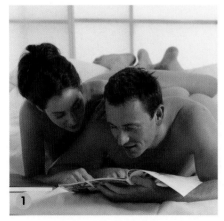

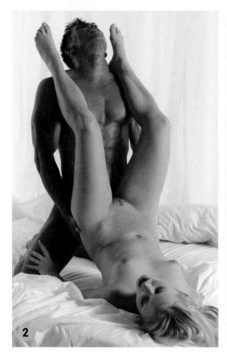

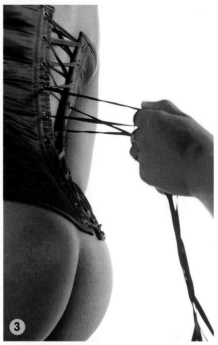

1 Erotica

Erotic literature can be a great aid to sex. It gives you access to your fantasies and often provides brilliant material to act out in the privacy of your bedroom. Why not present him with a poetry evening, accompanied by a tasteful striptease?

If you're turned off by tacky porn from the newsagents, try something with a little more class. Getting away from the hard stuff, there is a wonderful variety of sensual and erotic films that are guaranteed to get you in the mood – even reading a sex manual together can be inspirational.

At the other end of the scale, the gritty porn films and dirty magazines can have their own appeal because of their explicitness and lack of subtlety. Surprise him with an erotic video next time you are having a quiet night in – you might both find it thrilling to view something that appears so naughty, especially if you then try out the moves.

2 Anal sex

Most men find anal sex enjoyable, either penetrating a woman or being penetrated themselves – just name the ways.

For him, practising anal sex on a woman is a tighter and more intense experience. For you, if it is done correctly and carefully, the vaginal and rectal walls can swell during arousal, stimulating the G-spot and providing sensations that you could not get from vaginal penetration.

Men receiving anal sex from a woman with the help of a strap-on, finger or vibrator can have their prostate stimulated at the same time as she stimulates his penis. His G-spot, the prostate gland, can be accessed only through the anus, so it is an area that shouldn't be ignored.

The difference between anal pain and pleasure for either of you is relaxation. The keys to success are to keep clean, use plenty of lubrication and take it very slowly.

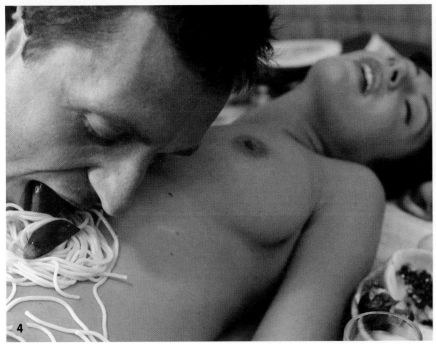

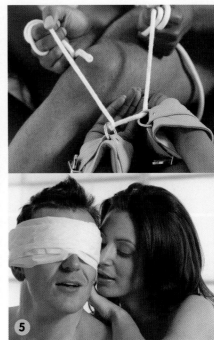

3 Dressing up

Dressing up and role-play are not just for drama students: you can re-create your bedroom as a dungeon of depravity, a hospital of hedonism or even Lara Croft's lair. It's an opportunity to put those fantasies into reality. You can buy outfits or make your own. Your boyfriend's a firefighter? Wear his uniform – it's bound to keep him smiling the next day at work.

You don't have to go to too much trouble, though. Most men find the old favourites – fishnet stockings and high heels – a turn-on, especially if you aren't wearing anything else. And the old-fashioned basque is sure to raise at least an eyebrow.

4 Feeding frenzy

Sex is meant to be fun. When you recognize that glint in your partner's eye, you will know that it's time to go and have a bit of adult play time. There are lots of games that

you and your partner can share to enliven the average bedroom romp, and not all of them have to involve his wearing your underwear. You could play naked Scrabble, but why not invite your man for dinner, with you as the first course? Cover your clean body with fresh fruit and cream, or seafood and asparagus, to really get him going. He can start at your toes, and work his way up to dessert. There are plenty of traditional aphrodisiacs that taste fantastic, whether they work or not. Sucking spaghetti off your stomach might be the only inspiration he needs. The list of food combinations is endless, whatever you fancy, but watch out if you are using anything hot or spicy in case it burns your skin or his tongue.

5 Bondage

We're not talking about sinister black masks, chains, long whips and complicated harnesses here. Although there are definitely

some people who love all that, there is also a lighter side to the scene, in which a larger proportion of people indulge. Bondage can be described as any sexual act that involves restraint, and it is important that it is consensual. Try tying his arms and feet to the bedposts, bedhead or even the banisters, using handcuffs (do remember where you put the key, though, as it will save considerable embarrassment later). Other materials include stockings, ribbon, silk scarves or his work tie – you can even buy special plastic tape that sticks to itself but is easy to undo. If you are feeling tentative, tie him up with tissue paper – fun, but also easy to escape.

He will be able to concentrate exclusively on his own sensations, without any feelings of guilt about his turn/your turn, and will love the feeling that you are in control. Some people who have difficulty achieving orgasm with penetrative sex find that a little light bondage resolves the problem.

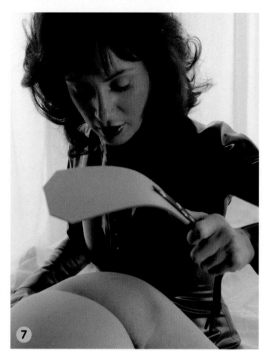

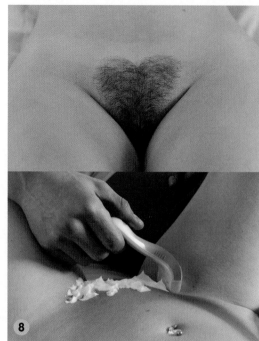

6 Masturbating for show

Watching their partner masturbate is one of the top five male fantasies. Yet the idea of masturbating in front of someone else, regardless of how much you may love and trust them, can be daunting. A good place to begin is to lie between your partner's legs, so that he can embrace you, but you do not have the sensation of being watched. As you get used to it, you will become bolder.

7 Spanking

Some men simply enjoy the odd thump on the rump. Remember to keep within your preset boundaries to prevent either of you from getting unintentionally hurt. In the heat of the moment, you may forget your own strength. Begin slowly and gently with a light slap or two, and then, if you want, increase the pressure in response to your partner. Keep it light-hearted and fun, and make sure you give as good as you get.

8 A bit of fun

Give your partner a surprise the next time he sees you naked. Many women wax or shave their pubic hair to keep it trim and tidy, but a variation on this is to shave it into fun patterns (or off completely) or even dye it for the total makeover. He might like to get involved and do the shaving for you.

9 Talking dirty

OK, so you don't want to sound like a sewer, but some men find naughty words very stimulating. It can take just one four-letter word to drive some men wild, but how you approach this will depend on your style. There's no point shouting "Fuck me harder" if he is just going to stop in his tracks to make sure he is in bed with the right woman. Boosting his ego is the way to go – a man who feels confident that he is a good lover will make a better lover, so it is also an investment in your own pleasure.

10 Teasing

Arousing your man with the lightest of touches can be fun for both of you. Stroking him with feathers, or letting your hair caress his skin, will have all those nerve endings jingling before long.

Ask your partner to lie down, then, starting at his feet, stroke, tickle and tease your way up his legs, circumnavigating his genitals, and continue until you reach the top of his head. Use feathers, wisps of fabric, and anything else you can think of that will stimulate his nerves. If you have long hair, let it fall on his face or neck, then move your head to and fro to give a stroking motion. It will feel delicious.

Once your journey around his body is over, it wouldn't be fair unless you now gave some attention to the parts you bypassed earlier. Again, hair, feathers and fabric will all feel wonderful against his penis and testicles, leaving him begging for more.

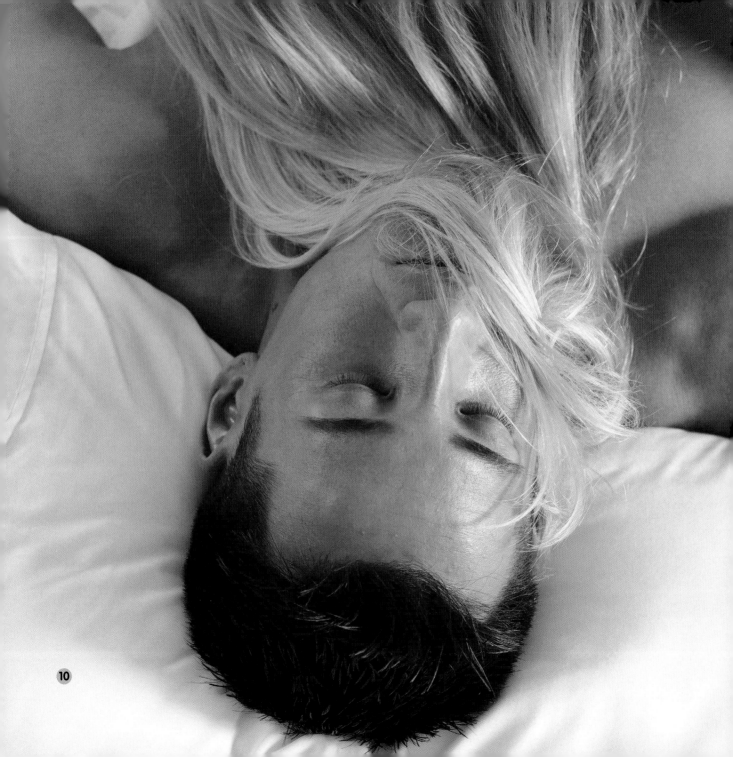

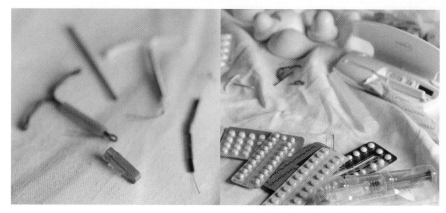

What every woman should know about contraception

Contraception and safer sex precautions should be paramount to everyone who has sex, not just people who do not want to have babies. Everyone should have been told about the importance of safer sex and should be well aware of the measures that can be taken, but for some reason too many people are still willing to take the risk of infection. Never assume that other people are as responsible with their bodies as you are. You have no way of knowing their previous history, and, in many cases, infection and disease are passed on unknowingly. Unprotected sex is never worth the risk.

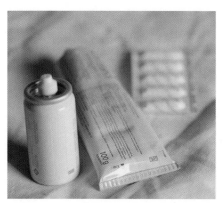

Hormonal methods
The contraceptive pill is hormone-controlled contraception, which is in the form of either the combined pill or the progesterone-only pill. The combined pill combines the two hormones oestrogen and progesterone to prevent the monthly release of an egg from the woman's ovary. If taken correctly, the combined pill is 99 per cent effective. It is not always suitable for women who smoke, or have conditions such as high blood pressure, circulatory disease or diabetes.

Barrier methods
Condoms, or sheaths, usually made of latex or rubber, are the most common form of barrier method. If used properly, they are 94-98 per cent effective, but always make sure they carry an official approval symbol.

Female condoms are made of quite thin polyurethane plastic. They fit inside the vagina and around the surrounding area, and, if used correctly, are 95 per cent effective. It is important that the man ensures that his penis enters the condom and does not get in between the condom and the vagina, or it will fail to protect.

The diaphragm or cap is another method of barrier contraceptive that is 92–96 per cent effective. It is a rubber dome that fits over the woman's cervix to prevent sperm from entering the uterus. It must be used in conjunction with spermicidal jelly or pessaries and should stay in place for six hours after sex.

Intrauterine methods
These methods of contraception fall into three categories: the intrauterine device (IUD), the intrauterine system (IUS) and the relatively new Gynefix. They all work in a similar way and are fitted, by a doctor, inside the uterus.

The IUD is a T-shaped plastic device that works by stopping the sperm from reaching the egg and preventing the egg from implanting in the uterus. IUDs can make periods heavier and more painful.

The IUS works in a similar way to the IUD, but contains the hormones progesterone and oestrogen, which are gradually released into the body. This system can reduce heavy periods and period pains and is over 99 per cent effective.

Gynefix works in a similar fashion to the IUD and IUS, except it has a more flexible frame. It is composed of a row of copper beads, which bend to fit snugly inside the uterus, and has a fine nylon thread attaching it to the uterine wall, so it is more secure and less likely to be expelled. It can also assist in relieving heavy and painful periods and has been shown to be more than 99 per cent effective as a contraceptive.

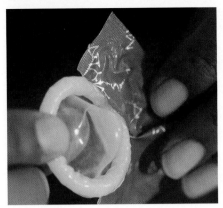

Natural methods

Using natural methods of contraception involves identifying the fertile days of the woman's menstrual cycle (the time from the first day of a period until the day before her next period starts) and abstaining from sex during these days. The fertile time is the time during ovulation (release of an egg). Although the egg will only live for about 24 hours, sperm can survive in a woman's body for much longer, up to seven days in some instances, so sex one week before ovulation could still result in pregnancy.

Noting the different signs of ovulation can be done by either using a hormone-testing kit, the temperature method or noting dates and cervical secretions. These methods are used as often by those attempting pregnancy as those seeking to avoid it and are more effective if the different methods are combined. The efficacy of these natural methods is cause of some debate – if in doubt, a barrier form of contraception should be used as well.

Permanent methods

Male and female sterilization are permanent methods of contraception that some couples opt for if they are sure that they do not want children or that they already have all the offspring that they want. They are not for people who may have doubts, however small, since they are usually not reversible.

How to use a condom

Sheaths are an effective protection against infection and are the most easily available contraceptives, but they have a reputation for creating clumsy pauses in lovemaking. One way to get around this is for the woman to put it on the man as part of foreplay. If you've never used a condom before, practise putting one on a banana.

The condom will come ready rolled in the packet. When you tear the packet, be careful not to tear the condom itself, or you will compromise its effectiveness. Place it over the erect penis, squeezing the bubble on top to exclude the air from it (otherwise the condom may burst later on), and simply roll it down. It should be put on as soon as the penis is erect, because semen can leak out before ejaculation. Although robust, they must be used with care as they can split or come off. Make sure he withdraws as soon as he comes and that he doesn't spill any semen.

Protect and survive

Semen has immuno-suppressant qualities. These are important for vaginal penetration, as they allow the sperm to enter the vaginal canal without being attacked by the woman's immune system. When sperm is swallowed, stomach acids break down these properties. Little is known about the effects they have in the anal passage, so it is important to use condoms when performing anal sex to protect against STIs such as HIV and AIDS. Anal sex without a condom can result in faecal matter and bacteria becoming trapped in the man's urethral opening. This can lead to infections in the man, and also in the woman if vaginal penetration follows anal sex. Thicker and stronger condoms are usually advised for use in anal sex.

Using lubrication or contraceptive jelly with condoms can help to prevent female urinary tract infections. Make sure you do not use oil-based products, however, as they reduce the effectiveness of condoms by 90 per cent: water-based lubricants are best.

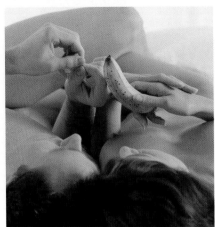

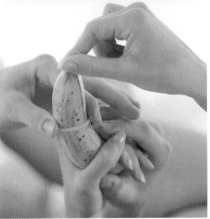

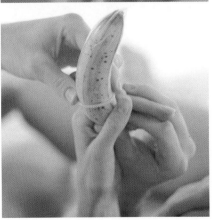

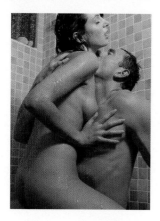
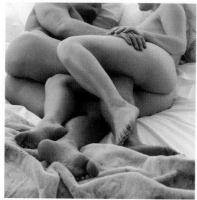
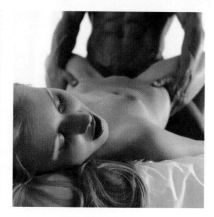

Index

AIDS 63
al fresco 29
anal beads 36
anal probe 19
anal sex 58, 63
Ananga Ranga 48, 50, 51, 52
anticipation 8
anus 17, 44
armpits 10, 14 , 15
ascending position 53

beaches 28
biting 51
blow-jobs see oral sex
bondage 59
bottoms 15, 17
butterfly kissing 13

calligraphy grip 19
Cleopatra's kiss 34
clitoris 22
cock rings 36–7
coitus 22, 58
    man on top 24
    rear entry 22, 27
    side by side 22, 26–7
    sitting positions 25, 26, 52–3
    standing positions 27, 53
    woman on top 22, 24–5
condoms 62, 63
contraception 62–3
crab embrace 52
cross 26

detour kissing 13
diaphragms 62
dildos 36, 37

domination 56
dressing up 19, 59

ears 10, 13, 15
elevators 28
embracing 50
erogenous ecstasy 36
erotica 48, 50–1, 58
Eskimo kissing 13

faking it 35
fantasies 56
feeding frenzy 59
feet 10, 14–15
fellatio see oral sex
fingers 10, 13, 14, 15
foreplay 17, 18–19, 50
foreskin 17, 43
French kissing 13
frenulum 17, 43
full frontal hugging 25

G spot see prostate
glans (head) 17, 32, 43
going down see oral sex

hair pulling 51
harness 37
hip rotator 26
HIV 63

ice-cubes 13
infection 62
Internet 56

Kama Sutra 48, 52
kama's wheel 52–3
kissing 10, 12–13, 50–1
    French 13

fingers 13

lovers' lane 28
lubrication 18, 37, 63

Malla, Kalyana 48, 50, 52
masturbation 17, 34, 35, 60
mile high club 29
mirrors 28
motels 29

navel 13, 14
neck, nape of, 13, 15
needs, meeting 7, 22
nibbling 13
nipples 15, 17, 34
noisy kissing 13

offices 29
oral caress 10
oral sex 7, 40–3, 52
orgasm 32, 33–4

pelvic floor muscles 34–5
penis 17, 32
perineum 17, 19
Pill 62
places for sex 28–9
placid embrace 53
prayer pumper 19
premature ejaculation 32
prostate 19, 34, 44, 58
pubic hair 51, 60
pushing the boundaries 56, 58–9

rimming 44, 56
rising dough 18
rising towel 35
rock and roll 35

rodeo ride 25
rubbing noses 13

San Francisco shuffle 19
Scrabble 59
scratching 51
sensation seekers 37
shopping spree 36
shower head 26
showers 29
silent kissing 13
simultaneous orgasm 34
skin-on-skin contact 26
soixante-neuf 45
spanking 60
spectator sport 35
squeeze 35
sterilization 63
stop and start 35
suspended congress 53

talking dirty 60
Tantric sex 32, 35, 48
tastes 43
teasing 60
testicle tantalizer 19
testicles 17, 32, 34, 44
thighs 15, 17
toes 10, 14
touching 14–15
toys 36–7
turn and twist 19

vagina 22
vibrators 36

wandering kissing 13
water 29
wrists 10, 15